THE MIRACLES OF MINERALS

The Human need for ninety plus elements
from a cell's point of view

by

Albert E. Carter

and

Larry Lymphocyte
(a cytotoxic T cell)

AIR Publishers
Provo, Utah 84606

Dedication

To family, friends, and fellow Citizens
and especially to my wife, Diane, who had the courage to
continue to encourage me even after her editing

Disclaimer

This book is for education only and should not be considered as
a substitute for consultation with a duly licensed medical
doctor. Any attempt to diagnose and treat an illness should
come under the direction of a physician. The authors are not
medical doctors and do not purport to offer medical advice,
although one of the authors (Larry) professes to know more
than both our doctors and our scientists.

Front cover:

    Floyd Holdman of Orem and Scitran of Provo

TABLE OF CONTENTS

INTRODUCTION

It is a disturbing experience to look in the mirror in the morning and see my father looking back at me. Especially since my father has been dead for over thirty years! That image looking back at me, the one I shave every morning is the way I remember my father appearing. But I don't feel that old. I don't think I could ever feel as old as my father appeared to me. In fact, I feel very young. At times I feel as young as I did when I was eighteen. Snap a good pair of skis on me and drop me out of an airplane on the top of a good ski run in the middle of the winter, or drop me on a good Nissen Goliath Trampoline any other time and I will show you how young I really am. Actually, there are only a few give-a-ways as to my chronological age. One of course is the mirror. Another is when one of my children accuse me of being too old fashioned. That hurts. That is what I used to say to my mother and father, especially when they would reminisce about the good old days.

"You are only as old as you feel," so goes the saying. Of course, those who are saying the saying are those who are older than what they would like to be. I have not started to say that yet. Well, I guess I have. I just did. But I don't make it a habit of saying it. You might say I am in denial, because I don't believe I am getting older. In fact, I am getting younger. Okay, okay. "That's impossible," I hear you say. And you are right if you are talking about chronological age. Every day I wake up I am one day older, but I am not aging. In fact, I appear to be ten years younger today than I did just one year ago.

Wait. Don't slam this book shut. Hear me out. Then decide for yourself if what I am telling you has merit.

About five years ago I was bouncing barefoot on a trampoline. This was nothing new to me. I was a professional trampolinist for twelve years and an amateur gymnast for twelve years before that. I am right at home on a trampoline. Anyway, a double back somersault was executed too low, so when I landed on the trampoline, I tore the toe nail off from my left big toe. This is an experience I would not wish on my favorite enemy. The pain was excruciating. The blood and gore was almost as bad. And it was down right embarrassing. After a couple of weeks of limping around, the pain finally disappeared, but the toenail didn't grow back, not the way that it should have. For some reason the nail would not adhere to the top of the toe so that it became necessary to cut it back almost to the quick. I lived the next four years without a toenail on the left big toe, something that you would never notice if you looked me straight in the eye, especially if I had my shoes on. My shoes also hid a pair of feet that were dry, callused, cracked and painful not only to me during the day but painful to my wife at night. Although she helped to relieve the problem by rubbing my feet with creams and oils, they were still dry, rough and cracked.

It was about this time that I noticed that the skin on my cheeks and across my nose was embarrassingly red and dry. A morning shower always ended with a moisturizing face cream after drying off with my bath towel. For the next four years I noticed that I could not stay in the sun too long because of the incredible sunburn to my face, which would then shed its skin like a snake.

It was two years ago that I began to notice the back of my hands. Something was happening. They were dry like an old man's hands and my forearms were so dry that when I brushed them with my hands the dry skin fell in flakes onto my pants like a snow storm. It was about that time, one morning, that my father in the mirror stared back at me and said, "Face it Carter. You are getting old. What do you expect? You are over half a century old. You are over the hill. From this time on its down hill to the grave. Nobody gets out of this life alive. Ashes to ashes. Dust to dust. You came from Mother Earth, and you will return to dust." I stared back at my father in the

4

glass and just stared. I had no argument. He was right. After all, I had already become him ... and he was dead.

"I need a rebounder," Dan Clark said, "but I would like to trade you these mineral supplements for it."

"Sure," I said. "You have been telling me about your great mineral supplements, so I would like to try them. I'll trade a rebounder for a supply." I felt it was a good trade and I was curious anyway. I took them home and began to take them daily. The first thing I noticed was the toenail. It began to stick to the quick. In less than two months I had a new toenail on the big toe of my left foot! Next, I noticed that the back of my hands became soft and supple. My dandruff disappeared at the same time that the pink dry blotches on my face cleared up. Now, I rub my arms and no snow storms! The bags under my eyes are gone and my close friends are telling me that I look ten years younger. And as long as they continue to tell me those kind things, they will continue to be my friends. Even my father in the mirror looks younger than he has in years. And that makes me smile. And he smiles right back. But even more exciting. My feet are now soft and supple so that I no longer feel embarrassed when I take them to bed with me.

These changes in my physical body are so dramatic that they obviously have my attention. Is it possible that one can reverse the aging process? Or at least slow it down? If so, how much? How long will it take? How much will it cost in time and money? Is it worth the extra effort? I'll never know unless I try.

CHAPTER 1

CONTACT

I had an idea where to begin searching for the secrets to longevity of life. There were several theories that were kicked around several years ago. At the time, they were so far out that I tried to forget them, but they wouldn't go away. These theories just continued to haunt me. Today, with my own rejuvenation happening, before my eyes, I decided it is time to explore them. If I am right, then Ponce de Leon wasn't wrong. He was just looking in the wrong place for the Fountain of Youth.

Obviously, this project is so important that I am going to need help, very special help. Those of you who have read The Cancer Answer are ahead of me. You already know who I am talking about. Larry helped me write The Cancer Answer in '87. If he is available, maybe he can be persuaded to help me with this project. After all even Larry has something to gain from this adventure. You see, If I am able to somehow live longer and healthier than expected, he could possibly live longer also.

You remember how I summonsed him the first time don't you? I certainly do. Actually it wasn't as painful as it sounds. Remember, I had the negative wire connected to a minute electrode implanted under the skin in my thigh just to the right of my right quadriceps? The positive wire was connected to a silver chloride electrode. My objective was to expand on Dr. Bjorn Nordenstrom's work where he used an electrical charge to destroy specific cancer cells. Then it happened. A little over an hour into the experiment, I heard, "Can . . . you . . . hear . . . me?" I remember that the voice was tiny and strange but very distinct. I also remember thinking that somehow I was picking up some radio transmission from across the campus. It was at that time that Larry the Lymphocyte made himself known to me. His voice was clear when the stethoscope I was using to monitor my heart touched the silver chloride electrode. Little did I know that out of that strange meeting would come a book of such magnificent quality and information that it would change the lives of thousands, even hundreds of thousands of people.

You know, after that first painful meeting it became easier and easier for Larry to communicate with me, and visa versa. The communication lasted until the book was complete, then it stopped. Sometimes I have dreams in which it seems Larry or something is trying to get through to me. That is why I think I should try to reestablish that communication again. However, the method of communication will be on my terms this time.

Chemistry is the physical science that deals with the composition, structure, and properties of substances and the transformations that these substances undergo. Because the study of chemistry encompasses the entire material universe, it is central to the understanding of other sciences. A basic chemical theory has been formulated by our scientists as the result of centuries of their observations and measurements of the various elements and compounds. According to this theory, and it is only a theory, matter is composed of minute particles called atoms. More than 100 different kinds of atoms are known and are called chemical elements.

I know this might be redundant for those of you who have excelled in chemistry and still remember what you learned, but it is important to lay a good foundation of understanding for those of you who may not have a strong background in Chemistry.

According to the theory, atoms of the same element or of different elements can combine together to form molecules and compounds. The atoms are held together by forces, primarily electrostatic, called chemical bonds. Notice the electrical implications even at the atomic level.

The study of organic chemistry originally was limited to compounds that were obtained from living organisms, or live things, while the study of inorganic chemistry included compounds derived from all of the elements except for live things. The study of the relationship of the two is called Biochemistry.

Recent research in tissue culture, physiology, and biochemistry has demonstrated a need for an all-inclusive compendium on minerals as well as vitamins and hormones. In addition, great interest has been generated in presentation of properties of the actual controlling agents which accurately blend all the cellular enzyme systems and organelles to produce a living cell, and from that a living multicellular organism. It is precisely in this area of control mechanisms that the minerals, vitamins, and hormones play such key roles, because they are the controlling agents.

Biochemistry is the subdivision of chemistry in which the compounds and chemical reactions involved in processes of living systems are studied. Now, to do this, scientists need exacting instruments to study minute changes in the substance being studied. In the laboratory, the most modern chemical instrumentation has three primary components: a source of energy, a sample compartment within which a substance is subjected to the energy, and some sort of detector to determine the effect of the energy on the sample. Frequently, the energy source is electromagnetic radiation. An X-ray diffractometer, for instance, enables the chemist to determine the arrangement of atoms, ions, and molecules that constitute crystals by means of scattering X-rays. Most modern laboratories contain ultraviolet, visible, and infrared spectrophotometers, which use light of various wavelengths on gaseous or liquid samples. By such means the chemist can determine the electron configuration and the arrangement of atoms in molecules.

In other words, we have been studying, investigating, poking, prodding and, spying on the internal environment of the cells of the human body without even asking for their help or even their permission. Of course, none of our scientists have ever thought of asking permission. Who or what would they ask anyway? And how would they ask?

This is where my theory begins to kick in. I have taken these ordinary earphones and converted them into a communicating transducer. In order to ask, we need to identify an entity to ask and have a method for asking. So, we need a transducer. Stay with me here. For you who don't know, a transducer is a device that transforms input energy into output energy; the forms of the input and output energy may be identical or different. The electric conversion transducer, for example, changes electricity from one frequency to another, and some of the most common transducers, like the telephone, change energy from one form, sound waves, into another, electricity. Now, get this. Atoms are held together by electrical bonds to form molecules, so all functions inside each cell are bioelectric. Enzymes, hormones, nerve messages are all bioelectric. Can you see where we are heading?

Let's take the low electrical conductivity of boron, an inorganic mineral, as an example. Its conductivity increases greatly as its temperature is raised. At certain temperatures, therefore, boron behaves as a semiconductor, and it is often added to germanium and silicon, two other minerals, to increase their electrical conductivity.

Research suggests that boron may be nutritionally important. Apparently, it helps to maintain appropriate body levels of minerals and hormones needed for bone health. Boron and possibly silicon and germanium, three inorganic minerals could possibly be used by the cells of the body for the very same reason we use them; as semiconductors in cellular communication.

Now, that is why I have altered these earphones. They are my transducers. You see, ultrapure germanium can be produced in near-crystalline perfection more easily than other semiconductors. The crystalline boron and silicon semiconductors have been added to these earphones so that they will be able to pick up any bioelectric transmission from within my head. Naturally, if this works we will have produced the very first real "<u>cell</u>-u-lar phone."

The earphones will not be used like a familiar electroacoustic transducer where the sound wave impinges upon a diaphragm inside causing it to move. The minute electrical energy coming from specific cells within my head, possibly magnified by the inner ear, will be picked up by the semiconductors inside the ear piece and electronically sent to my computer which I have altered to receive this form of communication. In other words, I will not be hearing anything, but my computer will. What it will hear I don't know exactly. But whatever it receives will be printed out on the screen.

In modern electronic computers the transistor is the device that acts as a switch. When computers using transistors were first built, the size of each transistor was about 1/8 square-inch. Today, hundreds of transistors can reside in a comparable space when integrated in a semiconductor chip.

Progress in semiconductor technologies continues, producing increased processing speeds and the fitting of more circuitry into less space. The latest attempts is the integration of thousands of circuits on a silicon wafer.

The products of advances in semiconductors give designers the freedom to build functions into hardware that previously had to be provided by software. The result of this is that computers gain both speed and versatility.

The ultimate computer, the human cell is still far beyond our most advanced designs, but like the human cell, the processes that are used to make microscopic integrated circuits are themselves made possible by computers. These technologies, like human cells, take advantage of the unique properties of silicon and other inorganic minerals to create not only transistors, but also complex conducting pathways and other elements within single, small chips.

The similarities between the operational function of the computer and what we are learning about the function of the cells of the body is enough for me to try to establish a link between the two communication systems.

A relatively new area for computers is that of communications from computer to computer, such as the Information Super Highway. Well, if communications consist of the flow and control of information, this is part of what a computer was designed to do. It manages the data moving among the elements within itself. That is also the scientific description of the enzymic activity inside each cell. Of course, there are major differences in that cellular communication is organic, was created by God and has existed since life began, while computer to computer communication is a creation of man; computers are inorganic. However, we are coming closer to computer/cellular communication. And when we create the link between the ultimate computer, the cell, and our manmade computers, gains in cellular/computer communication will provide an important breakthrough in understanding ourselves like never before.

The technologies and benefits that will be derived from this area of study will undoubtedly filter down to many areas of both health and computer science. Much work in cellular intelligence research will involve programs built to perform in ways similar to the ways in which humans are able to remain healthy. To an extent, this is a method for learning about ourselves from the inside out. But, despite certain advances in cellular intelligence, computers can still do no more than their programs instruct them to do. The greatest successes in this field will come with huge, database systems that act like expert consultants in such fields as health, medicine and chemical analysis.

So there you have it. The next step is to do it. All I have to do now is to plug my converted earphones into the computer and wait to see what happens.

Thursday. 19:36.

"I am sitting in front of my computer in the dark. Waiting. Nothing. This experiment started at 17:00 hours. I came into my office, turned on my computer, plugged the earphones into the serial port of the computer, sat down and got comfortable. I slid the transducers over my ears and here I am. For the first half hour, I closed my eyes and concentrated on sending a message to the inside of my body. The message was simple.

"I would like to communicate with you. Communication can be established at the inner ear."

All human cells are far more intelligent than we have thought until recently. Especially the cells of the immune system. Immunologist William Paul of the National Institutes of Health states, "The immune system is compared favorably with the most complex organ of them all, the brain. The Immune system has a phenomenal ability for dealing with information, for learning and memory, for creating and storing and using information."

It's an incredible system. It recognizes molecules that have never been in the body before. It can differentiate between what belongs there and what doesn't. I am counting on that ability. Just as this experiment is new to me, so also is it new to the white blood cells of my body. And we know so little about this incredible fighting force within. The field of immunology is progressing so rapidly that the medical journals are out of date by the time they are published.

"Communicate ... communicate ... communicate with me. Talk to me." I really feel funny sitting here in the dark with these funny earphones on. I'm glad that nobody can see me. "Communicate. Communication is possible at the inner ear."

Converting my computer was rather easy when I recognized that in order to process numbers and data electronically, it is necessary to represent information as numerical quantities. Of course, all data is coded as binary numbers (0) or (1). If six-bit sequences are used, then 64 possible characters and digits can be represented. But the nucleotides of the deoxyribonucleic acid (DNA) of the cells are trinary. However, the way the ribosomes read the ribonucleic acid (RNA) in groups of three to produce proteins means that there are only 64 possibilities. In theory, all I had to do is to match up the 64 binary possibilities with the 64 trinary possibilities and cellular translation, here we come!

"Talk to me. Communicate."

Another application of personal computers is in the area of electronic, or desktop, publishing. In this blossoming technology, software programs and inexpensive printers are used to produce text and graphics that are camera ready for publication. Sitting at a single terminal, a user can write and edit text, produce such graphics as charts or drawings, lay out text and graphical elements, and store the results in memory. The results can then be printed out or sent electronically to a typesetter. Desktop publishing allows individuals, even if they are only cells, to produce high-quality printed matter inexpensively. My objective is to establish cellular/computer communication and take it to the final step. Publish it. If it works, I won't have to type everything into the computer. It will already be there. So, although Larry the Lymphocyte will do the work, nobody will believe that this book actually came from a Cytotoxic T Cell. After all, who ever heard of a Cytotoxic T Cell writing a book?

Communicate ... comm... Wait. Something is happening. I feel a buzzing in my left ear. Now it is beginning to feel like an earache. There seems to be a swelling inside. White blood cells rush to the scene of an infection, like when a sliver or a thorn breaks the skin and introduces outside germs into the body. Maybe the white blood cells are rushing to the area of disturbance, which would be the inner ear.

Communicate with me. My computer is able to translate. My thoughts now intensified with the impending breakthrough.

Suddenly, something appeared on the VCR screen in front of me.

"~`~`""""~~~````"`.,.,.::`~~~````||||"

A message! The computer received a message! I will type a response. "Computer received message. Do not understand. Try again."

"~`~`""""~```""""`.,.,||"

I typed, "Our alphabet has 26 letters beginning with A and ending with Z. It begins, A, B, C, D...." Then the computer screen began to function like it had a life of its own.

"W e   k n o w   t h a t.   We are testi n g," appeared on the screen.

"Great!" I typed. "Then we can communicate!"

"W e   alw a y s   c o u l d.   Y ou   d o   not   w a n t   to   l iste n."

"Amazing! Do you realize what a breakthrough this is?" I typed.

"O f course. W h e r e do y ou t hin k you got t h e id ea s?"

"Well, they just came to me over a period of time."

"Y ou ar e re ce ptiv e , but n ot too cognizant."

My fingers flew over the keys as I tried to share my feelings. "My left ear seems to be warm, slightly painful, but more tingling than anything."

"W e assembled b y chemotaxis."

"What? You have taxis?" I asked good naturedly. "We have taxis too. That is how we get around sometimes."

"For your information, Carter, we have the ability to move by ameboid motion. That means we can move through tissue at speeds of up to 40 microns per minute. Chemotaxis is the ability of single cells to move towards a specific point in the body. In this case, your inner ear."

Now curiosity took over as amazement wained. I typed, "Who am I communicating with? Is Larry Lymphocyte with you?"

"Y e s ."

"Who? Which one of you is Larry?"

"We a r e Legion, for we ar e many."

"Yes. I can feel your presence, but where is Larry Lymphocyte?"

"We are . We h a v e divided into m any."

"Of course. I should have known. Old cells never die, they just multiply."

"Cells don't grow old. Peo ple d o."

"Corrected again. Larry, you haven't changed. It is great to be talking to you, all of you again. How many are you?"

"W e are L e g i o n . . ."

"Yes. I know, for you are many. Well, I guess, the more, the merrier."

"The more, the healthier, Professor Carter."

"Yes Larry, or should I say, Larrys?"

"Larry will do. We answer as one. Our DNA is exactly the same. We are what you would call identical twins many times over."

"Okay. Now that we've got that straight, what would you like to talk about?"

"Life."

"That's a big subject. Can you be more specific?"

"Yes. Your life, specifically. Your age in particular. You are getting older, meaning you are getting closer to death. If you die, we die."

"Larry, that is a question that has baffled man since time began. The Spanish explorer Juan Ponce de Leon, 1460-1521, is credited with the discovery of Florida. According to legend he was seeking the Fountain of Youth--a rejuvenating, tonic spring that Caribbean natives had described. He explored the Florida Keys and part of the west coast of the peninsula before returning to Puerto Rico by way of Cuba. In July, 1521, he was mortally wounded by an Indian arrow and returned to Havana, where he died. So he didn't find the secret of long life."

CHAPTER 2

LIFE

"Larry, there is every indication that almost all of us are concerned with both life and death ... especially our own. I am no exception. To me birth is very mystical and death is mysterious. And while I am alive it is my intention to separate the two events just as far as I can.

"Our life span denotes the length of time intervening between conception and death, during which we undergo remarkable changes in structure and function. In the embryonic stage the fertilized egg progressively differentiates into a highly complex multicellular organism. After birth we enter the juvenile phase, which is characterized by growth in size until sexual maturation, when growth slows down and eventually ceases completely. After the peak of the reproductive period, physiological capacities of various organs begin an inexorable decline, with a consequent increase in the probability of death.

"It is understood that all organisms have a finite and species-characteristic life span that reflects the underlying rates of aging."

"Are you sure about that?" The question appeared on the screen as I paused for a moment.

"Well, there is a tremendous variation in life span among different groups of organisms. Differences in the longevity of species, hybrids, mutants, sexes, and strains lend support to the view that life span is genetically determined."

"But is it?" Another question appeared.

"We know that life span is measured either as the maximum age achieved by a member," I continued, "or as an average among the population. The former reveals the genetic potential, whereas the average life span reflects the hospitality of the environment and is a more meaningful measure. The maximum natural life spans of various organisms range from about eight days in some to over one hundred fifty years in tortoises and over four thousand years in the bristlecone pine."

"Life span means different things to different individuals, then." I couldn't tell if that was a question or a statement. So I continued to type.

"We humans are the longest-living mammals and among the longest-living of all animals. The human's inherited potential life span is arbitrarily placed by some at 150 years..."

"Who set your life limit at 150 years?"

"Well, Larry, I don't know, because, as of 1990, the highest authenticated age was 120 years." I have had experience with Larry before and I could tell that he was leading the conversation the direction he wanted to take it. Most of the time I was pleasantly surprised when we reached the final conclusion.

"We do not understand old age because we do not age. Please inform us."

That I will try to do. In modern Western societies, old age, the final stage of life, is thought to begin at 65 or 70, although aging proceeds at different speeds in different people. In earlier societies, old age began sooner; people in their 40s were considered old. Because of advances in medicine and hygiene, and a softening of the rigors of life, many more people now reach the ages of 65 or 70 than did in the past.

"Oh, come on, Professor Carter. Give us a break. Aren't you going to give us any credit for keeping your ancestors alive longer?"

"Well, yes. I guess so, but advances in medicine and hygiene had a lot to do with it."

"You wouldn't have been able to do it without us."

"I guess not," I responded. I then continued, "In 1978 more than 24 million Americans were 65 years of age or older. The proportion of older people to the rest of the population has been increasing. In 1900 only 4% of the population was 65 or over; in 1970, the figure was 9.6%; in 1980, 10.5%, 1990, 11.2%; and demographers expect it to reach between 12 and 14% by the year 2000. This suggests that by 2030 one American in five will be 65 years of age or older.

"We want you to be one of those," the Larrys typed. *"We would like to show you how."*

"You will have no argument there. I am enjoying this life. But if you are going to show me how to live longer, you will have to show me how to be healthy the rest of my life."

"You leave that to us," appeared on the screen.

This is going to be an exciting adventure, I thought to myself.

"I hope so," flashed the screen. Then I remembered that Larry could read my mind, was aware of every thought and dream. Everything I studied was available to them. Yes, this was going to be an exciting adventure. I decided to go to the library and read up on the theories on aging, because I had a theory of my own.

CHAPTER 3

THEORIES ON AGING

"Okay, Larrys, let's see what we have learned," I typed right after I had placed my transducer earphones over my ears. Immediately the words began to spill onto the screen.

"Various theories of the aging process have been proposed. Among these are the environmental theory, the metabolic theory, the genetic theory, and the immunological theory."

"Great Larry, I knew you could do it. Look Ma, no hands." I folded my arms and read the screen as the words which I had read that morning appeared on the screen.

"The environmental theory of aging stresses the importance of the changes with age in the environment of the living cells. For instance, such deposits as collagen and calcium salts may accumulate, and in a number of organs-- including the thyroid gland, the gonads, and the muscles--the number of fibers and the bulk of fibrous tissue may increase. As a result, the epithelial cells often are living in a different and less favorable environment in old than in young individuals."

"Is that right, Larry?" I asked.

"Not exactly," came the reply. *"The environmental theory suggests that the deposits of collagen and calcium salts are inevitable."*

"And they are not?" I asked.

"No. Vigorous exercise to increase internal body fluid circulation, achieving proper chemical balance within the

internal environment and efficient enzymic activity will solve those problems."

"Interesting," I typed. "Continue."

"The metabolic theory of aging is actually a more scientific version of the old "wear and tear" theory, which says that the body of an organism--like many of the machines produced by humans--has a life span limited by the amount of daily use. According to this concept, a life of stress and overexertion, with inadequate time for rest and recuperation, is a deterrent to longevity."

"According to that theory, if I don't exercise I'll live longer."

"Quite frankly, I don't see how your scientists came up with that one. Your body is not some machine made by humans that wears out with use. It has the ability of improving with use. In fact, all the cells of your body have the ability of becoming better at what they do with proper use. However, overexertion, misuse, abuse of various parts of your body or even lack of enough rest may reduce the ability of any or all of the cells to recuperate. After all, we are only human ... cells, and as such we have to rely upon your common sense."

"Maybe a more recent extension of the metabolic theory suggests that the production of free radicals by damaged tissues, over time, causes future cell death."

"Carter, there is no doubt about that. Free radicals, chemical molecules inside your body that are not properly paired with other chemicals, will do whatever it takes to become paired with another molecule of any other element that has an electrical imbalance. They are like little bullets to otherwise healthy cells. But we cells have that condition under control, just as long as we can rely upon you to provide us with the proper nutrients, exercise and rest. We cells produce plenty of super oxide dismutase, a chemical that absorbs all of the free radicals created when cells die. But for some reason you humans don't appreciate that. In fact, you seem to be

doing everything to thwart our effort to protect you from the inside."

"What do you mean by that?" I asked.

"The air you breathe is not pure air. The water you provide to us is filled with too much chlorine and floride. It contains pesticides, insecticides and industrial chemicals. These kill cells by the thousands and each cell that dies produces hundreds of free radicals. That's a lot of extra work for us just to keep you healthy. It is vitally important for us to be able to control the onslaught of the free radicals," Larry continued throwing words on the screen.

"What can you tell me about the genetic, or gene-mutation, theory of aging?"

"Explain, please."

"During the life of a human, spontaneous mutations lead to an accumulation of errors in the control of gene expression that result, finally, in old age."

"You forget, Carter, that we human cells have the ability of living indefinitely. It is you humans who are dying. Our job as lymphocytes is to search and destroy mutant cells before they can become cancerous."

I folded my arms again after I typed, "Please continue."

"The immunological, or autoimmune, theory states that every cell in an individual organism is immunologically similar to every other cell in that organism. If cells undergo change from their genetic pattern, as occurs in mutation, the immunological character of those cells may change. Both nuclei and cytoplasm of such cells may produce substances known as autoantigens. Other cells react to autoantigens by rejecting and killing such cells or by walling them off by deposits."

As I read the words as they appeared on the screen, I could feel a burning sensation across the back of my neck. I knew what was about to happen, and it did.

"I cannot believe the ignorance of some of your scientists," I read. Larry was on a rampage. I could feel the temperature rising. I knew I had a fever. *"They are ready to blame the immune system any time they cannot come up with the right answers. We get the blame for Addison's disease, allergies, juvenile diabetes, multiple sclerosis, myasthenia gravis, rheumatoid arthritis and lupus. Your doctors would have you believe that we become confused and stop functioning, or actually attack the body's own cells. We are not traitors to the body. Our job is to protect, not destroy. They tell you this because somebody has to take the blame and until now we have not been able to talk back. Well, things have changed. We are going to tell the truth. We ..."*

"Hold on Larry. We will accomplish nothing by you getting me hot under the collar."

"All right, Carter. You are right. Sometimes human logic is good, I guess."

***

I've been doing a lot of thinking over the last few days since my reunion with Larry Lymphocyte, or should I say the Larrys, since there are obviously more than one. First, I should apologize to you. Larry has very little tolerance with people. Especially when it comes to misinformation about the human body. You see, he... they feel that they know more about the inner workings of the body than all the medical doctors and scientists combined, simply because the doctors and scientists are on the outside looking in and Larry is there on the scene. If there is an injury, the lymphocytes are there to make sure that no foreign invaders breach the wound until it is healed.

Actually, they are very protective of this body. And I do appreciate them for that.

I wanted to type that in here before I put on the earphones. I am sure Larry will have something to say about that. "Okay, Larry, the earphones are in place, the computer is turned on and tuned in. Speak, oh great macrophage."

"Is there a difference between chronological age and aging?"

"I suppose so. Chronological age refers to the passage of time; generally, when the question is asked how old a person is, the answer is given in units of time, say, years. We even celebrate the passage of years with birthdays."

"Yes, yes. Go on."

"You sound anxious, Larry. Is there a problem?"

"Yes, we are running out of time, or years."

"Physiological age means the health and physical condition of the organism in relation to chronological aging. Thus, you are only as old as you feel."

"So chronological age isn't important. It's the physiological age we have to work on."

"Yes. You can't do anything about chronological age, but physiological aging, or old age, is a widespread biological phenomenon that occurs in all higher organisms and in many of the lower ones. Its signs usually are a decrease in such functional capacities as the metabolic rate, the ability to sense and respond to stimuli, and the ability to move and reproduce. Aging organisms also have an increased susceptibility to disease, injury, and predators."

"Your old age is probably due to our inability to fully restore damage inflicted at the molecular level."

"Right. Aging causes some degree of physical and psychological change in everyone. With age, reflexes become slow, joints stiffen, and eyesight and hearing decline. By the age of 65, four people out of five have at least one chronic condition such as arthritis, heart disease, or atherosclerosis, although the condition may not impose any limitation on their main activities. However, both the extent and severity of health problems become greater as the person grows older. People over the age of 75 have more chronic conditions and higher rates of disability than do people between 65 and 74. Most cognitive processes, including perception, intelligence, and memory, decline with age. Although most older people retain enough psychological skills to function adequately, there is considerable variation among individuals in the effects of both physical and psychological changes."

"Al, what if we told you that we know a way to correct any damage at the molecular level and reduce susceptibility to disease, injury, and predators?"

"Well, our scientists tell us that moderate exercise, relaxed life-style, and balanced diet tend to prolong life, whereas smoking, excessive drinking, and mental stress shorten the life span.

"You didn't hear us, Carter. Wake up. This is your body speaking. We are trying to communicate with you. While it may be statistically convenient for you to think of people over 65 or 70 as "old," there are of course many exceptions. Some are caring for parents of their own, who may be in their eighties or nineties; a few are still active in business or politics."

"Well, our scientists tell us that dietary supplements such as vitamins or drugs have not as yet proven to have any significant beneficial effect on the rate of aging."

CHAPTER 4

THEORIES ON DEATH

"You are not reading your terminal, Carter. We know a way to overcome old age and death for you."

"Larry, the size of the body is genetically limited and when growth ceases certain changes set in. With increasing age come changes in the genetic components of a certain number of somatic (body) cells. These changes may be marked aberrations in the size and shape of the cell nuclei and nucleoli, abnormalities of chromosomes, and the occurrence of irregular cell division. The nucleic acid DNA may incur permanent lesions, especially in the liver."

"Carter, you are like all other humans. You don't want to blame yourself for your short life span so you blame us, the cells of your body. We are keeping you alive and healthy right now. Where is your faith? We have already proved our ability to keep you healthy haven't we?"

"Of course, Larry, and I thank you for it, but we age primarily because the cells of the body, especially those which cannot replace themselves, undergo changes that result in decreased function, degeneration, and death. Don't you agree?"

"When you are right, I agree. However, the different kinds of cells vary markedly in their ability to replace themselves. Such as surface layers of cells (epithelia), those which form the outermost skin and the lining of the digestive and other tracts are able to replace themselves rapidly. Red blood cells are constantly generated in red bone marrow, as are white blood cells in such lymphoid tissues as the lymph nodes, the thymus, and the spleen."

"No argument there. However, the nervous system, has generally irreplaceable cells known as neurons. Changes in human neurons, and the loss of these cells, occur in all parts of the human brain. Although the disorder atherosclerosis may greatly increase the rate and severity of neuronal changes, such changes occur independently as part of the aging process. Cells of the heart, the voluntary muscles, and certain parts of the immune and endocrine systems also cannot be easily replaced."

"We agree that those cells need to be protected more than those which can replace themselves, but that is not an impossible task if you know how."

"And if you are healthy yourself, you can do your job more efficiently. Immunological changes with age are those which involve the defense mechanisms, especially those that fight against bacteria, viruses, and other foreign substances."

"Right. Your cellular defenses consist of the white blood cells, including lymphocytes, neutrophils, some phagocytes that devour bacteria and others that produce antibodies."

"During the aging process certain immune functions decrease with age, while the incidence of cancer, of immune diseases, and of infections increases."

"Yes, that is the way it is now, but it doesn't have to be that way, big buddy."

"Oh, how are you going to stop the hormonal changes which profoundly affect the functioning of the body? The most apparent change is the decreased production of sex hormones, producing the onset of menopause in women and certain changes in men. Among other changes, lowered levels of insulin occur, causing increased risk of diabetes mellitus."

"We agree that humans are a more complex organism, but your health is still dependent upon us. The healthier we are, the healthier you are. Agreed?"

"When you are right, I agree, however, because we are more complicated, the stage in which changes occur in the functioning of the nervous system, especially of its higher centers, is termed senility. It is difficult to differentiate senility from old age. Changes in gait, for example, may be due to changes in the nervous system or to changes in joints, ligaments, or muscles. Senility is probably a distinctive condition, not just an acceleration of the normal aging process. Personality changes are common in senility, as are the onset of paranoid tendencies and fits of irritation or depression."

"We think we are glad we are not human."

"I see you still have your sense of humor, Larry. That is good."

"Professor Carter, we have been communicating about old age, a condition we hope to be able to show you how to avoid, but that is just a condition before death. We want to be able to help you postpone that also. Death is so final."

"Larry, nobody gets out of this life alive. Death is the cessation of life resulting from irreversible breakdown of respiration, or the process by which most organisms use oxygen to produce the chemical energy supporting life. Death may result from physical injury, disease, or deterioration caused by aging. It may occur at the level of cells, tissues, organs, or the entire body."

"Yes, we understand death more than you realize. We are killers of bacteria and viruses. We destroy fungi. We eat dead cells to keep you clean of metabolic trash around the tissue spaces. We see death every second. That is why we feel you should listen to us."

"Higher organisms die gradually, beginning with the cells and tissues and progressing to organs and then the entire body. In humans the irreversible arrest of heart action was once viewed as the only conclusive proof that life had ended."

"That is because when the heart stops beating, the cells of the body are deprived of oxygen and die; the brain cells are the first to die, suffering irreversible damage when they are

31

without oxygen for 5 to 8 minutes; the kidneys can function up to 1 hour, the striated muscles for hours, and such parts of the body as nails and hair for days."

"I see you do understand death.   In humans, the definition of death often includes the cessation of circulatory and cerebral function (brain waves) as well as the cessation of respiratory function.

"I guess I will never really understand the human race. They make a simple thing like dying complicated."

"Complicated and sometimes expensive. Records of the cause of death in the United States indicate that most deaths are the result of chronic diseases such as heart disease, cancer, or diabetes mellitus, in which death is anticipated over months or years. Most Americans die sometime after reaching 65 years of age; it is estimated that the average dying person spends about 80 days during the last years of life in a hospital or nursing home. Life is often prolonged at the expense of great suffering and indignity to patients and their families. Larry, we have been communicating about old age and death. It is not very uplifting. I was hoping to write about something more enlightening; something that would lift the spirits of our readers."

"That's great.   That means we are still heading the same direction.   We have just dug the trenches for the foundation. Now it is time to form the foundation."

"Oh, you know how to build houses also?"

"You have been planning one for sometime now.   We can read your mind like you read a book.   We have been paying attention to the details. By the way, when you get ready to build, check with us.   We have a few suggestions for the internal environment."

"I'll bet you do. Look, if you can't swing a hammer, I don't need your suggestions."

"That's all right. We will still be there for repairs when you smash your thumb."

"Thanks."

THE MIRACLES OF MINERALS

CHAPTER 5

IN THE BEGINNING

The buzzing in my head was getting stronger as I reached my office. A splitting headache, actually. It started the first thing in the morning. That's how I awoke. Under other circumstances, I would have taken an aspirin, but I knew the source of my pain and I also knew how to end this misery. I could hardly focus on the keyhole as I fumbled for my keys. I stumbled through the doorway, and poked at the "power on" switch of the computer. I grabbed the earphones and slid them on at the same time I was sitting down in front of the computer. "Come on. Boot up." I said between my teeth. It didn't speed things up, but it did make me feel better.

"The earliest forms of life known are bacteria-like cells dating back to 3.5 billion years ago," came scrolling across the screen.

"How life was originally formed, however, is open to controversy," I typed back. "Various creation accounts dating back thousands of years attempt to explain how life began. A version well known in the western world is the biblical account by which God created the world, then plants and animals, and finally the first man and woman. Many people consider creationistic views to be correct and believe that life is so complex that it must have been formed by Divine intent. Also, many believe that each form of life was created in the beginning and did not evolve from lower to higher forms of life."

"The Greek philosophers Anaximander and Aristotle promoted the theory of Spontaneous Generation--that life constantly arises from nonliving organic matter--for the origin of life."

"This theory was put in doubt by the work of the Italian physician Francesco Redi (1668) and the Italian scientist

Lazzaro Spallanzani (1776)," I rebutted, "and discredited by the French chemist Louis Pasteur (1861)."

"The British naturalist Charles Darwin developed his theory of the evolution of the species in the 19th century," scrolled Larry. *"The scientific community came to accept Darwin's theory, in modified form."*

"I know, Larry. Numerous scientists have since attempted to explain the initial development of life. In the 1920s, the Russian biochemist Aleksandr Ivanovich Oparin and the British geneticist J. B. S. Haldane, suggested that certain organic chemicals present in primitive oceans combined to form self-reproducing forms, a reaction that was aided by an atmosphere rich in hydrogen. This chemical soup theory was tested in 1953 when the American chemists Stanley Lloyd Miller and Harold Clayton Urey, created a model of a primitive environment in their laboratory. Under these conditions, Miller and Urey were able to produce amino acids and other biologically important compounds."

"Carter, there were scientists who suggested that life reached Earth by means of spores from outer space."

"Researchers, however, have found various forms of amino acids on meteors, which could be taken to support this concept. In addition, in the 1970s a team of Canadian and English scientists developed the Life Cloud Theory. It states that organic chemicals present in stellar dust clouds could react to form nucleic acids and proteins, which then settle on a planet to form living organisms."

"That still does not answer the question of how life began."

"Don't get so excited, Larry. Does it make any difference how life began? I mean let's concentrate on how to live longer and healthier. Life exists. Let's enjoy it as long as we can."

"Your scientists think they know everything."

"They are only human, Larry. Give them room to explore and discover."

"Carter. Can't you see that they are taking too long? We need this information in your life time to do us any good."

"Well, you now have the ability to communicate. Maybe you should consider helping them."

"That is exactly what we have planned in our DNA."

"I kind of figured that. So don't let me stand in your way. You have access to the computer. Let's see what you can do?"

"The quality known as life is generally easy to recognize but has been difficult for biologists to define."

"Why is that?" I queried.

"Living forms--microbes, plants, and animals--have the properties of metabolism, growth, and reproduction. Many also move and respond to external stimuli."

"Agreed."

"Nonliving objects can have some of these properties, but by no means are they considered to be alive."

"Like viruses?"

"Exactly. Viruses cannot reproduce by themselves. They have to rely on the use of the DNA of living cells in order to reproduce."

"So, Larry, tell me, what are the characteristics of living things?"

"Living material consists chiefly of the elements carbon, hydrogen, oxygen, and nitrogen. Metabolism is the ability of living forms to combine food and oxygen in order to obtain energy for their normal function. Plants, blue-green algae, and some bacteria produce oxygen by using light energy through photosynthesis. Certain lower organisms known as anaerobes cannot use oxygen but instead depend on other chemical pathways to obtain energy."

"So, let me see if I understand what you are saying. The cellular biology may be presented as a set of six statements:

(1)   all living material is made up of cells or the products of cells;

(2)   all cells are derived from previously existing cells; most cells arise by cell division, but in sexual organisms they may be formed by the fusion of a sperm and an egg;

(3)   a cell is the most elementary unit of life;

(4)   every cell is bounded by a plasma membrane, an extremely thin skin separating it from the environment and from other cells;

(5)   all cells have strong biochemical similarities; and

(6)   most cells are small, about 0.001 cm (0.00004 inches) in length; for example, the smallest cells of the microorganism mycoplasma are 0.3 microns in size, whereas some giant algal cells may be several centimeters long.

"Now I know why they call you Professor, Professor."

"What does this have to do with health and longevity?"

"Most organisms start life as single cells, you call zygotes, and grow into massive multicellular bodies, like you, with cells of considerable differences in form and function."

"This process, which involves growth and differentiation, is called development."

"Although skin cells, liver cells, brain cells, and so on, are highly differentiated, they are all derived from the original zygote as a result of the high-fidelity copying of DNA during mitotic division. This is achieved by a complex, little-understood process whereby different genes are active in different tissues. Individual cells in multicellular organisms, like you, normally die as part of the developmental sequence. During the development of vertebrate limbs, for example, cell death and resorption shape the digits, thighs, and upper arm contours."

"Yes, I know, little buddies. Recent experiments by our scientists indicate that cells taken from animals and cultured in the laboratory also have a finite life span, and that death is an inherent property of cells themselves. Cultured normal embryonic cells undergo a finite number of population doublings by division and then die."

"That is the current understanding of your scientists, but do you realize that bacteria and other unicellular organisms that reproduce asexually rather than sexually continue to divide indefinitely and thus cannot be said to age?"

"Yes. We had this discussion in The Cancer Answer."

"Any bacterial cell divides to produce two young cells; thus, division for such organisms is a process of rejuvenation. Protoplasm, the living substance that makes up both the cytoplasm and nuclei of cells, are potentially immortal. Within the phylum Protozoa, organisms that consist of a single cell, are numerous species that reproduce by fission and have real or potential immortality."

So, if I have this straight, you want to be able to live indefinitely."

"If we were not part of your mortal body, we could. Even Dr. Arthur C. Guyton in <u>*Medical Physiology,*</u> *states, Each of the 75 trillion cells in the human being is a living structure that can survive indefinitely and, in most instances, can even reproduce itself, provided its surrounding fluids contain appropriate nutrients."*

"You've presented a good, well documented argument. I guess I need to know more about my 75 trillion cells. "From your point of view, then Larrys, what are the components of living organisms?"

CHAPTER 6

PROTEINS

"All organisms capable of independent life (in other words, all except the viruses) are made principally of fats, proteins, carbohydrates, and nucleic acids."

"When we think of protein, we think of beef, chicken, or some other animal products. From your point of view, what are proteins?"

"Proteins are polymers of smaller molecules, the amino acids."

"Okay, so what are amino acids?"

"Amino acids are organic compounds that are the building blocks of proteins. In most animal metabolisms, a number of amino acids play an essential role. The genetic code, which determines the assembly of amino acids into body proteins, is mediated by the nucleic acids."

"Well then, tell me about nucleic acids."

"One thing at a time Al. Let's understand amino acids first. In terms of structure, each amino acid has at least one carboxyl (COOH) group, which is basic."

"Did you know that the name of the acids comes from the stem word amine, meaning *derived from ammonia*?"

"That doesn't surprise us, Carter. Ammonia is a by-product of protein digestion. Amino acids don't come from ammonia."

"I know, but our scientists didn't know that when they were naming things."

"Amino acids join together in long chains, the amino group of one amino acid linking with the carboxyl group of another. The linkage is known as a peptide bond, and a chain of amino acids is known as a polypeptide. Proteins are large, naturally-occurring polypeptides. Many different amino acids are found, but only about 20 of which are the main constituents of human proteins."

"Only about half of these amino acids are classified as essential nutrients, that is, necessary in the human diet," I added.

"That is because we know how to manufacture at least half of them. Actually, we know how to manufacture most of them but not in large enough quantities for you to remain healthy without you supplying them in your diet."

"Are these amino acids different from each other?"

"Although all amino acids have amino and carboxyl groups, they all differ in the rest of the molecule."

"So, the shape and overall properties of a protein are dependent upon its constituent amino acids."

"Yes. In some proteins, a change in just one amino acid in the polymer chain, out of a total of perhaps 250 amino acids, or even a change in its position, can cause the protein to become nonfunctional."

"Wow, I didn't realize that. What do you mean, nonfunctional?"

"If it is an enzyme, it might perform its function differently or not at all."

"Wait a minute, I thought we were talking about proteins and amino acids. Now you throw the word, *enzyme* into the conversation."

"Look Carter, your chemists are currently trying to relate the role of each of these amino acids to the way in which the protein works, but that may take another ten or twenty years and we don't have that much time to waste. A major part of all enzymes are proteins and proteins are made up of amino acids."

"Okay, so let's talk about enzymes just as soon as we understand proteins."

"Have it your way. You are the professor. Proteins are an essential substance in the diets of humans and most animals because of their constituent amino acids."

"You've made your point. Please continue."

"Nutritionally, complete proteins are those which contain the right concentrations of the amino acids that we cells cannot synthesize from other amino acids or nitrogenous sources. So Carter, an adequate diet may be achieved by consuming a correct mixture of fruits and vegetables containing many proteins, some of which might be deficient in one amino acid but rich in another."

"I will study what I eat to make sure I am doing that. And if I am, what will you do with these proteins?"

"A first step in the digestion of proteins is their cleavage by protein-splitting enzymes into smaller chains of amino acids, or peptides. These initial peptides are then cleaved into smaller and smaller peptides until free amino acids are available. The amino acids are absorbed from the intestine by a complete biochemical process and are circulated by the blood to the cells that utilize them. Some of the amino acids are used directly as the building blocks in the synthesis of new proteins unique to the needs of that part of the body. Others may be used to supply energy, and still others, particularly when large amounts of proteins are consumed, may be excreted in the urine."

"You do know your job, Larry."

"Oh, its far more complicated than that, but it is hard to keep the explanation simple enough for humans to understand."

"In addition to the 20 common amino acids, are there other amino acids?"

"Yes. Others occur in proteins from plant and other animal sources. There are about 25 to 30 amino acids used in other proteins. In addition, more than 50 amino acids, not combined in proteins, have been found in plants. Some of these are simple derivatives of the common amino acids; others, usually found in plants and microorganisms, have more complicated structures."

"So how do you get from the amino acids, the building blocks of proteins, to the construction of proteins?"

"That is a very good question, Carter. We have the answer because all of the proteins your body will ever need are manufactured right inside the cells of your body. And the nucleic acids DNA and RNA are the keys that link amino acids together to form proteins. Proteins in the form of enzymes, in turn, regulate the formation of carbohydrates and fats."

"Please explain, oh great intelligent amoebas, step by step, for us ignorant humans, just how you construct all of the proteins for the human body."

"The genetic material DNA is copied, or reproduced, and passed on from parent to offspring."

"We did that without your help."

"Your offspring begin life as fertilized eggs. The offspring are never entirely identical to their parents because they acquire half the genes from each parent and also because

of slight errors in passing on the parents' hereditary information."

"Is this leading to protein synthesis?"

"Yes. The process of protein synthesis within the cells is crucial for life because the proteins play essential roles in all aspects of cellular function. For example, proteins serve as enzymes (biological catalysts), structural components, hormones, and antibodies."

"Do all cells manufacture proteins?"

"Yes. A bacterial cell may contain the information for 2,000 to 4,000 proteins."

"Wow, that's a lot!"

"We human cells are able to produce 50,000 proteins."

"I'm impressed. I have a hard time baking a cake!"

"We know. You have fed the end results to us. The genetic information in all cells is contained in the chemical sequence of the deoxyribonucleic acid (DNA) of the cell. Similar to information stored on a computer tape, the genetic information in the DNA of the cell is of no value unless it is retrieved or, to use a biological term, expressed, by the cell. The term, gene expression, refers to the complex process by which the cell uses the genetic information in the DNA to synthesize proteins."

"So this computer work is old stuff to you?"

"We've been doing more complicated computer synthesis for thousands of years. We have had to wait for you to develop your simple binary computers so that we could share with you some of our secrets of life. Now may we continue?"

"Oh, sure, don't let me stand in the way."

"I believe you are sitting."

"Yes, Larrys, you little munchkins, when you are right, you are right."

"Please don't interrupt. We will be as brief as possible, but in order to understand how genetic information is used, the structure of DNA and proteins must be examined. The DNA molecule is a long, double-stranded polymer composed of four nitrogen-containing nucleotide bases--adenine (A), cytosine (C), guanine (G), and thymine (T) - a sugar, and a phosphate segment of the DNA that contains the information for one protein is called a gene. The amino acids form the basic unit of all proteins. Twenty different amino acids are available to form the long protein chains."

"Where are these amino acids found?"

"They are loose in the cytoplasm inside each cell. A typical protein may consist of 200 to 400 amino acids, linked by peptide bonds. In the genetic code, or triplet code, each set of three nucleotide bases in a DNA molecule contains the information for one amino acid. The sequence of these nucleotide bases determines the sequence of amino acids in the protein.

"Many steps are involved in the overall process by which the information in the DNA is used for protein synthesis. These reactions require another nucleic acid: ribonucleic acid, or RNA. RNA differs from DNA in that it contains a different type of sugar; also, one of the nucleotide bases of DNA, thymine, is replaced by another base, uracil (U).

"In the overall process of gene expression, or protein synthesis, the DNA, which contains the genetic information for a specific protein, is used as a template to make messenger RNA (mRNA). This "rewriting" of the genetic information is called transcription. The mRNA is then used by the cell to direct the synthesis of proteins in the process of translation.

Two other types of RNA are needed for translation of the mRNA: transfer RNA (tRNA), which is involved in going into the cytoplasm and finding each of the 20 amino acids and delivering them into protein; and ribosomal RNA (rRNA), which is associated with the ribosomes--organelles that are located in the cell's cytoplasm."

"What are Ribosomes?"

"Ribosomes are the site of protein synthesis. The enzyme responsible for transcription and for the synthesis of all RNA in the cell is DNA-dependent RNA polymerase."

"There you go talking about enzymes as if they are magic. What are they?"

"Let's just say that they are like factory workers inside the cells. In the meantime, it is important for you to understand that enzymes are necessary to produce proteins. Three RNA polymerases exist, and all are present in the nucleus of the cell. These enzymes are polymerase I, which is located in the nucleolus and responsible for the synthesis of the ribosomal RNA; polymerase II, which is present in the nucleoplasm and necessary for mRNA synthesis; and polymerase III, which is also present in the nucleoplasm and is required for the synthesis of tRNA.

"In order to understand better the process of protein synthesis it is useful to examine the RNA species in more detail. As mentioned, the mRNA contains the genetic information originally in the DNA. This information in the mRNA is also in the form of a triplet code; that is, every three nucleotide bases (called a code word or codon) contain the information for one amino acid. The sequence of these bases in the mRNA determines the eventual primary sequence of the amino acids in the protein to be synthesized. Are you following this, Carter?"

"Barely."

"Specific triplet code words in the mRNA also tell the cell where to start the synthesis of a new protein and when the protein is completed. Usually the codon AUG, a triplet of adenine, uracil, and guanine, initiates protein synthesis, and UAA, UAG, or UGA signal the termination of protein synthesis. In the bacterial cell an mRNA molecule may carry the information for more than one protein. In contrast, a typical animal mRNA molecule generally codes for one protein only.

"Although the mRNA contains the genetic information for the amino acid sequence in a protein, somehow the amino acid must recognize that information. This crucial step in protein synthesis requires another RNA, tRNA, which has a dual function: it must interact both with the amino acid to be inserted into the growing polypeptide chain and with the genetic information on the messenger RNA for that amino acid. A typical cell has many tRNA species, all of which are able to recognize specifically 1 of the 20 amino acids. Transfer RNA interacts at one end with an amino acid while it can recognize the genetic information on the mRNA for that amino acid at another site, the anticodon region.

"It is important to note that the linking of the amino acid to the tRNA requires a specific enzyme for each of the 20 amino acids. These enzymes, known as the aminoacyl - tRNA synthetases, are crucial for the fidelity of protein synthesis, because if the wrong amino acid is linked to the tRNA it is possible that the incorrect amino acid eventually will be incorporated into protein. This error would change the protein, sometimes to the point that the protein no longer functions effectively during metabolic processes.

"The third type of RNA involved in genetic expression is ribosomal RNA. Ribosomes from all species are composed of two subunits, one large and one small. Both subunits contain RNA and proteins, but the size of the RNA and number of proteins differ in the subunits. The synthesis of proteins in the cell actually takes place on the ribosome bound to the mRNA. Many of the antibiotics that are known to affect bacterial growth inhibit protein synthesis by interacting specifically with

the bacterial ribosome; two examples are streptomycin and tetracycline. At the start of translation the ribosomal subunits in the cell bind either near one end of the mRNA or close to an initiator codon within the mRNA, which signals where to start the synthesis of a protein. During this process a specific species of aminoacyl - tRNA (tRNA having an amino acid linked to it) interacts with the ribosome-messenger complex. Once this initiation reaction has taken place, elongation of the protein chain can occur. In this process the ribosome moves along the mRNA, and the protein chain is synthesized, one amino acid at a time. Each amino acid that is incorporated into the newly synthesized protein is first attached to a specific tRNA before it is carried to the mRNA - ribosome complex.

"After the aminoacyl - tRNA is bound to the mRNA - ribosome complex the amino acid is linked to the growing polypeptide chain by the formation of a new peptide bond. The ribosome then moves along the mRNA to the next code word, which permits another aminoacyl - tRNA to bind to the mRNA - ribosome complex. Thus the genetic information (codons) on the mRNA determines the order by which the amino acids are added to the protein.

"During the synthesis of the protein, the protein remains attached to the ribosome until all the amino acids have been placed in the peptide chain. When the protein is completed a specific codon on the mRNA signals the cell to release the polypeptide from the ribosome. After the peptide is released the ribosome comes off the mRNA, dissociates into its subunits, and the whole process can begin once again."

"Whew. That's heavy reading!"

"That is as simple as we can make it, but you must understand that all cells of your body know and use this information continuously. Now that you understand proteins you are ready to understand enzymes."

"Before we do that, I would like to ask a few questions."

"Please, be our guest."

"Genes of the DNA control the structure of proteins, which are the main structural and catalytic molecules in an organism; hair, muscle, skin, tendons, and enzymes are all made up of proteins, right?"

"Yes. The order of the nucleotide bases in DNA dictates the corresponding order of amino acids that give proteins their specific shape and function during protein synthesis."

"So what is the real relationship between the DNA and a gene?"

"In humans, the DNA in each cell contains about 3 billion base pairs, distributed among 22 sets of autosomal chromosomes and one set of sex chromosomes in the nucleus. If all of this DNA were stretched out, it would have a length of about three feet, but the DNA is tightly compressed into the chromosome."

"Is all of the DNA considered genes?"

"Only about 2 percent of a person's DNA forms the actual genes. The rest constitutes either noncoding "spacer" regions between genes or noncoding "intron" regions within genes."

"I knew that."

"Sure you did, Carter."

"One more question. Please explain a mutation at the cellular level for me."

"Easy. We deal with mutations every day. A mutation is the process by which genes change from one form to another. Mutations may be caused by such mutagens as X

rays, ultraviolet rays, nitrous acid, ethyl methane sulfonate, and nitrosoguanidine."

"Then I should stay away from those as much as possible."

"Please do. It makes our work much easier. However, mutations are not always your fault. They may occur spontaneously as a result of accidental changes in the chemistry of the cell. Because mutation is a random, haphazard change, most mutants contain damaged genes that are nonfunctional. Mutants usually do not live long. A mutation in DNA usually results in an altered nucleotide sequence, either by substitution, addition, deletion, or insertion, which is translated into an altered amino-acid sequence that usually produces a change in the organism's normal body function. The alteration of amino acids can have a drastic effect on function, as in the case of sickle-cell hemoglobin. A mutation of the chromosome by transposition, translocation, or insertion can cause similar effects. Mutations of cells other than sex cells are a primary cause of cancer."

"Does this happen often?"

"All humans carry quite a large number of deleterious and lethal mutant genes that are recessive."

"So each mating is a kind of a lottery, in which the offspring reveal whether or not the parents' mutations are at an identical location."

"You could say that. If both parents are heterozygous for a gene pair in which the recessive gene is deleterious, then one-fourth of their children will show genetic disease of the kind controlled by that gene."

"Thank you, Larrys, ... all of you."

THE MIRACLES OF MINERALS

CHAPTER 7

ENZYMES

It is hard on my ego to be put down by a group of cells ... even if they are my own. It is rather revealing to me to realize that the most sincere, intelligent, best equipped scientist can only discover that which is already there. The complicated protein synthesis still is not completely understood by the best scientists we humans have to offer, but is common knowledge to all cells of the body."

"There is hope for you, Professor Carter. And if there is hope for you, there is hope for us."

"Thank you. It is a pleasure being instructed by such a magnificent team of experts."

"We do not argue with truth. What is catalysis?"

"What?"

"Come, Al. We don't have time."

"Well, the defining property of all catalysts is that they increase the speed of a chemical reaction without being used up or appearing as one of the products of the reaction."

"Good. Now we are ready to discuss enzymes."

"I was expecting this so I did a little research alone."

"You are never alone."

"You were obviously aware that I was diligent in my research, then?"

"You are to be commended in your effort. Please share with us what you found."

"Before the end of the 19th century, chemists understood that molecules must obtain extra energy before they can interact. The extra energy, or energy of activation, may be supplied when one molecule collides with another, or it may be supplied by an external source of energy, such as heat or ultraviolet radiation. The primary barrier to interaction, therefore, is the energy of activation, which is sometimes called the energy barrier."

"That is good, Carter. Please continue."

"The higher the energy barrier, the fewer the molecules that will pass over it, and thus the slower the rate of the reaction. The catalyst can then participate in the reaction again and again."

"Excellent, now if the word catalyst is replaced by the word enzyme, the fundamental enzyme catalysis is the result. In forming the complex, enzymes reduce the activation energy, or energy barrier, for a biochemical reaction. Enzymes are far more effective than inorganic catalysts in reducing activation energies; thus, they permit biochemical processes to take place at temperatures compatible with life.

"A nonbiological catalyst catalyzes a wide variety of chemical reactions. Enzymes differ from inorganic catalysts in two important ways: the sequence of amino acids in an enzyme molecule is specific to that enzyme and essential for the molecule's catalytic action; and each enzyme exerts its action only on specific substances in specific reactions.

"I also found that the term, *enzyme*, is derived from the Greek and literally means "in yeast" or "leavening." It was originally coined in 1878, when it was generally but erroneously believed that the yeast enzymes responsible for fermenting wine could function only in living cells. A leading biochemist of the period, Louis Pasteur, was a proponent of that belief."

"Once again your scientists were wrong."

"I know, Pasteur and the rest were proved wrong in 1897, when Eduard Buchner showed that enzymes isolated from yeast cells were capable of fermenting sugar to ethanol (alcohol) and carbon dioxide. Buchner's work is a landmark in the history of biology, for it ushered in a new era of biology in which most functions of cells have been shown to occur--and can be studied--in the test tube.

"In 1926, James Sumner first isolated an enzyme, urease, in crystalline form and showed that it was a protein.

"It is about time."

"Biochemists thereafter realized that the solution to the mysteries of enzyme structure, and how that structure promotes catalysis, lay in unraveling the chemical structure of proteins. Toward this end enormous progress has been made in recent years through the development of procedures for the isolation and crystallization of other enzymes."

"They should have asked us. We make them."

"Be patient with us, Larry. We are moving as fast as we can. After all, the first enzymes that yielded clues to structure and function were the protein-digesting enzymes chymotrypsin, trypsin, and carboxypeptidase, and the DNA-splitting enzyme ribonuclease. The first enzyme for which the entire amino-acid sequence has been elucidated is pancreatic ribonuclease. It is a protein containing 124 amino-acid units in a linear sequence. Although the amino acids are lined up end to end, various forces within the molecule cause it, like almost all proteins, to take the shape of a badly tangled ball of yarn."

"That is so we can store them in a small area inside the cells. The three-dimensional tangling, or folding, of an enzyme is called its tertiary structure. The information required for the correct folding is contained in the amino-acid sequence, which is dictated by the information encoded in the DNA. The

catalytic activity of an enzyme is determined largely by its amino-acid sequence and tertiary structure."

"So the cells of the body produce enzymes. Why are enzymes so important any way?"

"Metabolism, Carter. Metabolism is the sum of all the chemical reactions in the living cell that are used for the production of useful work and the synthesis of cell constituents. Almost all cellular reactions are catalyzed by complex protein molecules called enzymes, which are capable of speeding reaction rates by a factor of hundreds to millions. Enzymes serve to accelerate, or catalyze, the chemical reactions of living cells. Without enzymes, most biochemical reactions would be too slow to carry on life processes. The manufacture of these enzymes is regulated by the DNA through protein synthesis. The potential of a cell to grow and divide is determined largely by the number and different kinds of enzymes it contains. Certain cells also perform specialized functions, such as transmitting nerve impulses or producing hormones, that are regulated by enzymes. Several hundred different reactions may proceed simultaneously within a living cell, and each is catalyzed by one or more enzymes."

"Oh, I see, carbon dioxide gas is generated from bicarbonate when a bottle of soda is opened. The same chemical reaction occurs just before air is exhaled from the lungs."

"Almost, oh great body. The uncatalyzed reaction that occurs with a soda bottle, fast as it may seem, would be too slow to sustain life if it occurred in the lungs. The lungs have an enzyme that hastens the reaction. Similarly, without enzymes it might take millions of years for amino acids to spontaneously link together to form protein molecules. All cells, however, contain enzymes capable of catalyzing the synthesis of thousands of protein molecules in a second."

"I can see that a lot of work goes on inside each cell."

"Yes. We are constantly building things up and tearing things apart. Many structures in the living cell are of great complexity and periodically must be replaced. This process of building new molecules is called anabolism. Structures that are worn out or no longer needed are broken down into smaller molecules and either reused or excreted; this process is called catabolism. Great quantities of energy are required not only to produce the work needed for the pumping of the heart, for muscular contraction, and for nerve conduction, but also to provide the chemical work needed to make the large molecules characteristic of living cells. Anabolism and catabolism are aspects of overall metabolism, and they occur interdependently and continuously."

"Enzymes are made up of protein molecules, then?"

"Many enzymes contain, in addition to their protein part, a much smaller, nonprotein group called a coenzyme."

"And what are coenzymes made of? I know this, but I want you to explain this to our readers."

"Coenzymes are made up in part of individual vitamins and/or minerals and are essential for enzymic activity. The vitamin niacin, for example, is part of a coenzyme for several different enzymes concerned with the uptake of oxygen by cells." One-fourth to one-third of all enzymes involves a metal ion as a required participant."

"Right again, Larry. Our scientists know the uses of only a few of the trace minerals. But scientists do know that they are necessary for the work of such bodily compounds as enzymes and hormones."

"A coenzyme that remains firmly bound to the same enzyme during catalysis is called a prosthetic group; one that migrates is called a carrier. Pyridoxal is a typical prosthetic group, lipoic acid a typical carrier. Coenzymes participate in two important metabolic processes in living cells: biosynthesis, *or the building up of cell constituents; and energy utilization, or the burning of substances as fuel for energy."*

"So folic acid is a coenzyme essential for growth while acetyl coenzyme A is active both in the burning of carbohydrate and fat as fuels for energy, and in the synthesis of fats?"

"You got it, Carter. The most important coenzymes of energy metabolism are nicotinamide adenine dinucleotide (NAD) and nicotinamide adenine dinucleotide phosphate (NADP), which contain a derivative of the vitamin niacin."

"Why is that, dear Larrys?"

"NAD accepts electrons from the oxidation of biological fuel molecules and transfers them to oxygen. It functions primarily in the generation of the super energy source adenosine triphosphate (ATP)."

"That's the super bioelectric fuel all cells need to carry on their daily activities, right?"

"That is right, big buddy. NADP plays its most important role in photosynthesis: it is reduced in the light reaction and participates in carbon dioxide reduction in the dark reactions. And that is how it happens in plants."

"An *Enzyme*, is a protein molecule that speeds up chemical reactions in all living things. Without enzymes, these reactions would occur too slowly or not at all, and no life would be possible," I summarized.

"Right, and all living cells make enzymes, but enzymes are not alive."

So, enzyme molecules function by altering other molecules."

"Enzymes combine with the altered molecules to form a complex molecular structure in which chemical reactions take

place. The enzyme, which remains unchanged , then separates from the product of the reaction."

"Enzymes thus serve as catalysts."

"Yes. And a single enzyme molecule can perform its entire function a million times a minute."

"That's fast!" I exclaimed.

"It has to be." The Larrys returned. "The chemical reactions occur thousands or even millions of times faster with enzymes than without them."

"So, the human body has thousands of kinds of enzymes."

"Each kind does one specific job. Without enzymes, a person could not breathe, see, move, or digest food."

"So our very existence is dependent upon enzymes."

"You could say that."

"I just did. But we know so little about enzymes."

"You don't have to, as long as we cells do. Even Photosynthesis in plants depends on enzymes, but the plants don't have to know about enzymes, because the plant cells do."

"Many enzymes break down complex substances into simpler ones. Others build complex compounds from simple ones. Larry, this information is amazing."

"Most enzymes remain in the cells where they were formed, but some enzymes work elsewhere in the body."

"Are you telling me that some enzymes commute to work?"

"I guess you could say that. For example, the pancreas secretes the enzyme lipase, which travels to the small intestine to break down fats."

"Why haven't our scientists told us these things?"

"They are just learning for themselves. Besides, enzymes are too tiny to be seen even with the most powerful light microscopes."

"However, scientists must know through various research techniques that enzymes occur in a number of shapes and sizes. Although enzymes of different plants and animals have different protein structures, they do function in similar ways." ·

"You got it, but although enzymes are proteins, some must be attached to certain nonprotein molecules in order to function. Many of these nonprotein molecules are metals, such as copper, iron or magnesium."

"They occur as trace elements."

"They are part of the organic and inorganic compounds called coenzymes. If a coenzyme is tightly attached to the protein part of the enzyme, the unit is called a prosthetic group. Neither the coenzyme nor the protein part of the prosthetic group can function alone. Many coenzymes consist of vitamins, and or minerals."

"So, if a person's diet lacks adequate amounts of these vitamins, or minerals the enzymes cannot function properly, and various body disorders may develop."

"Humans know these as diseases which eventually leads to death. If you humans would cooperate with us, we would be able to keep you healthier by creating the right enzymes when needed."

"What do you mean by that?"

"The action of many drugs created by your scientists has been produced for the purpose of inhibiting or activating particular enzymes."

"I don't believe that."

"Antibiotics inhibit a variety of enzymes necessary for bacterial growth, but they also inhibit a variety of enzymes in the healthy cells also."

"Vitamin B_2, or riboflavin, activates a portion of the cell's enzyme-catalyzed uptake of oxygen; and vitamin C, or ascorbic acid, activates enzyme-catalyzed reactions involved in the manufacture of bone and connective tissue."

"Nerve gases, on the other hand, produce paralysis by inhibiting the enzyme that promotes the action of acetylcholine, which is necessary for the transmission of nerve impulses."

"How do enzymes work anyway?"

"The formation of the enzyme-substrate complex depends on a special relationship between the surfaces of the two substances. You could think of it as a template, or key-in-lock; that is, the enzyme contains a certain sequence of atoms called the active site, and only a particularly shaped substrate can bind to the enzyme at that site. The binding of substrate to enzyme causes the enzyme to curl and twist in a conformational change; this brings about the contact between enzyme and substrate necessary to catalyze the reaction."

"This concept is often called the induced fit theory."

"We cells must possess the means of regulating both the kinds of metabolic reactions that are to take place at any given time and the rates at which the reactions should occur."

"Oh, and how do you control the metabolism of the body?"

"Through controlling the amount of activity of enzymes."

"And how do you do that?"

"Such control may take one of three forms: induction of enzyme synthesis; feedback inhibition of enzyme activity; and proenzyme activation."

"So that we humans can understand how you cells control the metabolism, lets take each method one at a time. First, enzyme induction."

"Bacteria can vary their enzymatic composition widely. The specific enzymes required for utilizing a given nitrogen or carbon source are usually produced only during growth in the presence of that compound. Thus, the presence of the sugar lactose "induces" the bacteria Escherichia Coli to synthesize the enzyme beta-galactosidase, which permits these bacteria to use the sugar as fuel for energy."

"I understand. What is enzyme repression?"

"The repression of enzyme synthesis is when the addition of amino acids generally causes cells to cease forming the several enzymes necessary for producing those amino acids."

"In other words, the end product of a series of metabolic reactions, or pathways, evidently plays a special role in regulating the synthesis of the enzymes of its own pathway."

"We couldn't have said it better. This mechanism is more precisely the end-product repression, and it involves complete shutdown of the DNA-directed synthesis of the enzyme in question."

"Thank you, now describe feedback inhibition for us."

"In feedback inhibition, as in end-product repression, the end product of a metabolic pathway may block the activity

of enzymes in the same pathway. But inhibition involves the inactivation of enzymes, not the cessation of DNA-directed enzyme synthesis. When the end product reaches a certain concentration, it decreases the rate of its own synthesis by preventing the previous synthesis of substances necessary for its manufacture. The inhibitory action occurs when the end product binds with a previous enzyme in the pathway and so alters the shape of the enzyme as to inactivate it."

"You do know your business, Larrys. Finally, what is proenzyme activation?"

"Enzymes may be produced in an inactive form called a proenzyme or zymogen and activated only when they are needed."

"Could you give us an example?"

"Easy, Thrombin, for example, is an enzyme that causes blood to clot by catalyzing the conversion of the soluble protein, fibrinogen, to the insoluble fibrin; but blood normally contains the inactive precursor of thrombin, prothrombin, and clotting occurs only when prothrombin is converted to thrombin."

"I can see why this is necessary. Blood has to flow freely as long as it is inside the blood stream, but if there is a leak, the blood has to be stopped by clotting at the leak."

"Human intelligence never ceases to amaze us."

"Cut the sarcasm, smarty pants."

"We don't wear pants."

"I didn't mean ..."

"We know what you mean. That's another example of human intelligence at work."

63

"It appears to me that if some of the enzymes aren't working properly that some pretty serious symptoms would begin to appear."

"Now you are beginning to get the picture. A number of diseases involve an inherited abnormality in one or more enzymes. For example, Phenylketonuria is a deficiency of the enzyme phenylalanine hydroxalase, which causes an accumulation of substances that produce brain damage and severe mental retardation.

"A deficiency of the enzyme glucose-6-phosphate dehydrogenase can cause a breakdown of red blood cells when any one of a large number of drugs is ingested.

"Tay-Sachs disease is an enzyme-deficiency disorder that leads to early neurologic deterioration.

"Albinism is due to a lack of the enzyme tyrosinase. And in the muscle disorder known as McArdle's disease, there is a lack of the enzyme glycogen phosphorylase, which is concerned with supplying the energy for muscle contraction."

CHAPTER 8

HORMONES

We hear of men searching for the secrets of the ages which include good health, longevity of life, and peace of mind. In these searches, men have climbed the highest mountains and crossed the deepest oceans. We have asked many gurus and meditated for centuries. We have tried to get close to our innerselves and inquired of our spirits. We pray to God for health and strength. Yet we accept death when it comes and even blame death upon God. Is it possible that many of the answers we seek are right under our noses? I mean literally. The cells of our body know many of the answers we are seeking. All we have to do is ask and wait for an answer. For this reason I have come to the earphones converted to a transducer and connected to my computer. In this way the very special cells now identified as Larry Lymphocyte, a very familiar part of my immune system will be able to communicate directly to the computer. The communication will show up on the CRT. I have been able to ask questions by typing them into the computer. I have been amazed at the information the cells have available and are willing to share with us. I will now put the earphones on and ask a question.

"Oh great and intelligent Cytotoxic T Cells of the Immune System, speak to me and provide me with the secrets of the ages."

"Who are you trying to impress, Professor Carter? Do you not know that we can read your very thoughts before you can utter them? Know you not that typing such garbage avails you nothing?"

"That's easy for you to say. I've been telling some of my friends that I have been carrying on a conversation with some of the most intelligent cells of my body and all I get is a strange look. Even you must admit that this form of communication is unique."

"Unique, yes. But only in this time sequence. There will come a time when the human race will have advanced far enough that cellular communication will be commonplace. Then men will live to the age of a tree."

"Okay, little buddies, you have helped us understand how enzymes work, now fill us in on the hormones of the body."

"Sure thing, oh great organic monolith. Hormones regulate cell metabolism either by changing our membrane's permeability to extracellular substances or by altering the activity of intracellular enzymes. Groups of enzymes are linked together in so-called metabolic pathways (chains of reactions), and hormones often act by increasing or decreasing the activity of "pacemaker" enzymes that control major pathways."

"Sounds like traffic cops to me."

"More like chemical messages sent to the enzymes and the enzymes are intelligent enough to act on the message. For example, glucose uptake by muscle cells is controlled by the permeability of the cell membrane to glucose and by the enzyme hexokinase which catalyzes the phosphorylation of glucose to glucose-6-phosphate. Glycogen synthesis is controlled by the enzyme glycogen synthetase; glycogen breakdown to glucose, by the enzyme phosphorylase; and fat mobilization from fat deposits, by the enzyme lipoprotein lipase."

"Those are strange names, Larry."

"We did not name them. Your scientists did. We are using your language to communicate because you would not understand ours. The hormone insulin increases glucose uptake by muscle cells and increases the storage of glycogen

and triglyceride, and roughly matches protein synthesis to protein losses."

"Do all cells produce hormones?"

"Good question. All cells know how to produce all hormones, but only certain cells in certain organs are given the responsibility to produce certain hormones. They are so potent that they have to be tightly controlled."

"What are hormones made of?"

"Any of a number of chemical substances. A hormone is produced in one part of an organism, but it causes an effect in a different part. Thus, hormones serve as a means of communication among various parts of an organism. They act as chemical messengers that help the body function in a coordinated way."

"Obviously, you know all about hormones, but humans didn't always know. In 1902, scientists found the first definite evidence of the existence of hormones. That year, British researchers discovered that a chemical substance controlled certain activities involved in digestion. Since then, scientists have identified more than 30 hormones produced by the human body."

"I was wondering when you were going to contribute to this book, Carter."

"Most hormones in the human body are produced by organs called endocrine, or ductless glands. The major endocrine glands include the two adrenal glands, the pituitary gland, the four parathyroid glands, the sex glands and the thyroid gland."

You are right as far as you go, but a few hormones are produced by endocrine tissue present in organs that are not primarily endocrine glands. Such organs include the stomach and the pancreas."

"I didn't know that."

"You don't have to because we do."

"May I continue?"

"Please do. We will stop you when you are incorrect."

"Where were you when I took anatomy in college?"

"Where we have always been. We suffered through that experience also because we knew the answers and could not tell you."

"The endocrine glands secrete hormones into the blood, which carries them throughout the body. After a hormone arrives at its target, the organ or tissue it affects, it causes certain actions to occur."

"Actually, the hormones do not aim for a target. All cells have access to all hormones when they are released into the blood stream. But some cells are programmed to react to certain hormones at certain times. Let me give you an example. When you receive an advertisement in the mail for tires at 25% off, do you always go out and buy tires?"

"No."

"When do you buy tires?"

"When I need them."

"If you received an advertisement in the mail to buy tires at 25% off when you needed them, would you act upon that advertisement?"

"Probably."

"How many people in your neighborhood do you think received the same tire advertisement?"

"All of them, I suppose. I get it. The hormones are distributed throughout the entire body by the bloodstream and those cells ready for that particular hormone acts upon the chemical message."

"You amaze us, Carter. You are so smart, you should be a Lymphocyte."

"No thanks. I am having a hard enough time being a mere human."

"Hormones regulate a variety of body functions. They may be grouped according to the functions they control. These functions include the way the body uses food; growth; sex and reproduction; the regulation of the composition of the blood; the reaction of the body to emergencies; and the control of hormones themselves.

"Metabolic hormones regulate the various steps of metabolism, the process by which the body converts food into energy and living tissue. For example, the endocrine tissue of the stomach and small intestine secretes a number of digestive hormones. These hormones control the secretion of digestive juices, which break down food into simple substances that can be used by the body. After molecules of digestive food enter the bloodstream, other hormones, control their use by the cells of the body. For example, the hormones insulin and glucagon, both secreted by the pancreas, regulate the amount of sugar available to the cells. Insulin enables cells to use sugar from the blood. If the pancreas secretes too little insulin, a serious condition called diabetes mellitus results. Gulcagon causes the liver to release additional sugar into the blood.

"Two hormones produced by the thyroid gland, thyroxine and triiodothyronine, control the rate at which the cells use food and release energy."

"What would happen if the hormones were not controlled properly?"

"Overproduction of these hormones results in many physical and emotional disturbances; including excitability, muscular weakness, rapid pulse and respiration, and weight loss. Underproduction causes such symptoms as low body temperature, mental and physical sluggishness, and weight gain. By controlling the production of energy, these hormones regulate the way in which the body uses food in building new tissue. Thus, they play a major role in the creation of new proteins by the body cells.

"Other hormones also control the way cells use food to build new tissue. The glucocorticoids are a group of hormones that function primarily in regulating the metabolism of carbohydrates (sugars and starches), fats, and proteins. They control the processes by which the body converts digested proteins into carbohydrates and fats. These hormones include corticosterone, cortisol, and cortisone. The glucocorticoids are secreted by the cortex (outer part) of each adrenal gland. Insulin and growth hormone (GH), a hormone secreted by the anterior lobe (front part) of the pituitary gland, also regulate the creation of new tissue."

"You know, when we hear the word hormone, we usually think of growth and sex hormones."

"That is because most humans are preoccupied with sex and how big they are. The body's development from infancy to adulthood involves a complex process of physical changes. Hormones play a key role in regulating these changes. Growth hormone controls overall growth during childhood. Faulty production of this hormone during childhood can cause a person to become a dwarf or a giant. In adults, growth hormone enables certain tissues to maintain their proper size and structure. Insulin, glucocorticoids, and thyroxine also play major roles in tissue growth and maintenance.

"The sex hormones regulate the remarkable changes that occur during puberty. They help trigger a person's rapid growth in height and weight and, at the end of puberty, they stop this growth."

"Thank you for filling us in on hormones, Larrys."

"We cells have been filling you in all your life, Carter."

THE MIRACLES OF MINERALS

CHAPTER 9

ELEMENTS

"Larry. Larry. Do you read me? You usually are so anxious to communicate that you give me a headache. I have some questions I would like to ask all of you. You have helped us understand enzymes inside the body and what hormones are. But you left us with a major question. I would like your opinion about minerals. You indicated that enzymes need minerals. Which ones and how much of each?"

"You are aware that if it were not for the minerals in the earphones, we would not be able to communicate with your computer, right?"

"Right good buddies, but I only used two. What other minerals do you use, and for what reason?"

"Tell me Carter, what do you know about the elements of the earth?"

"Well, the concept of an element as it is understood today did not develop until the 17th century. In the days of the classical Greek philosophers Plato, and Aristotle, the material world was considered to be composed of four or five fundamental substances, or *elements*. Empedocles named earth, air, fire, and water as elemental substances, and Aristotle added ether, a perfect substance of which heavenly bodies are composed.

"These elements are not really material substances, Carter."

"I know, but they were idealizations of material substances. The qualities of temperature (hot or cold) and moisture (wet or dry) were attributed to each of the four classical elements. Fire, for example, had the two adjacent qualities hot and dry."

"And that, Professor Carter, is one of the reasons why humans do not live very long. Lack of vital information. Elements are simple indivisible matters which provide the primary components for the human body. They cannot be subdivided into newer components. It is from their combination that we cells are able to form other things."

"That means that there is hardly a difference between the ancient and modern concepts of elements."

"Surely you don't believe that do you, Carter?"

"Well, several actual elements were known to ancient civilizations. Gold, and to a lesser extent silver and copper, were found in their uncombined or elemental form in nature, and have been used as pure metals since 3,000 BC and probably earlier. The ancients also made iron, tin, lead, mercury, copper, and silver by reducing their ores to their elemental forms by smelting, often with carbon in the form of charcoal. In fact, the chemical symbols of all of the metals known to the ancient world are derived from their Latin names:

gold is Au from aurum,

silver is Ag from argentum,

iron is Fe from ferrum,

tin is Sn from stannum,

lead is Pb from plumbum,

and mercury is Hg from hydrargum.

Sulfur and carbon, two nonmetals found uncombined in nature as solids, were also known to the ancients. Many large sulfur deposits are found at or near the earth's surface. The ancients referred to sulfur, as well as other inflammable substances, as brimstone, and vast quantities of native sulfur are still mined for the production of inorganic chemicals such as sulfuric acid. Carbon is found in nature as diamond, graphite, and, in a less pure form, charcoal."

"You just explained how mankind related to many of the elements, but that is not how cellkind relates to them."

"Cellkind? I never heard of cellkind."

"There are a lot of things you have never heard of."

"Oh, I don't know about that. I keep up on scientific discoveries and writings."

"That is what we mean. Your knowledge is based on what your scientists tell you."

"I see nothing wrong with that."

"Oh yeah. Tell us, Carter, what are the necessary minerals for your good health?

"The major minerals occur in the body and are needed in large amounts. Calcium, phosphorus and magnesium are some examples."

"And the minor minerals?"

"Trace minerals are not called minor minerals because they are too important to be considered lesser elements."

"Very good, Carter."

"Since they only exist in very tiny amounts, or in traces, they are known as the trace minerals. Even the trace minerals are necessary to the proper functioning of the human body."

"Spoken like a true human scientist."

"Iodine is an example of a trace mineral. Very little is needed, but it is still necessary. Here is one approximate scientific analysis of the body's chemical-mineral content:

ELEMENT	PERCENTAGE
Oxygen	65
Carbon	18
Hydrogen	10
Nitrogen	3
Calcium	2
Phosphorus	1.1
Potassium	0.35
Sulfur	0.25
Sodium	0.15
Chlorine	0.15
Magnesium	0.05
Iron	0.004
Manganese	0.00013
Copper	0.00015
Iodine	0.00004
Cobalt	undetermined
Zinc	undetermined

And others not yet clarified.

"The ionic properties of trace minerals are used in both plants and animals in the enzymic activities inside the cells. In fact three trace elements - iron, zinc, and copper stand out as a distinctive subgroup with many ramifications. These three metals have been recognized as essential for over 60 years and are required in milligram quantities to implement multiple catalytic and other functions. They have attracted so much research that each has earned separate volumes. The remaining trace elements, a more numerous but less ubiquitous group, are utilized in submiligram or even microgram quantities."

"Since enzymes can be thought of as factory workers made up of proteins, some vitamins and minerals, and are responsible for all of the chemical reactions inside the cells,

how many minerals do we cells need to make the proper enzymes?"

"Are you asking me how many different minerals there are in the body?"

"Yes. We know, but do you?"

"Well, there are 15 mineral elements which consist of 5 macro or bulk essential elements, calcium, magnesium, sodium, potassium, and phosphorus; and 10 micro or trace elements, iron, copper, manganese, zinc, iodine, selenium, molybdenum, chromium, cobalt, and fluorine. Not all of the latter have been proved essential for <u>life</u> of man, but they have been proved essential for some living systems or for normal health and longevity in humans."

"How many minerals are needed for our enzymic activity?"

"I don't know. Let's see, there are literally thousands of enzymes participating in food digestion and metabolic functions of cellular growth and metabolism. And each enzyme needs certain vitamins and/or minerals to be able to do its very specific job. One researcher made an investigation and found 98 distinct enzymes working in the arteries, each with a particular job to do."

"Carter, how long have your scientists known about enzymes?"

"In 1930, 80 enzymes were known; in 1947 200; in 1957, 660; in 1962, 850; and in 1968, science had identified 1300 of them. Today there are well over 2,000 and climbing rapidly the closer we are able to look inside the cell."

"Just because your scientists didn't know about the thousands of enzymes in 1930, does that mean that they didn't exist?"

"Of course not. That is silly."

"We agree. Then, is it possible that more enzymes will be found?"

"I should hope so. With the passage of time, our knowledge about the number of elements present in the human body has considerably increased. Twenty years back we knew of only 19 elements in the body. Now, we know about 90 such elements. Therefore, it will not be proper to classify any element to be absent from the human body. And with the increase in knowledge about how the body uses the elements, I am sure that new enzymes will be identified."

"Then is it possible that your scientists will learn about how we utilize other minerals than the fifteen you mentioned?"

"Of course. On the basis of present ongoing research, it is most likely that selenium, molybdenum, manganese, chromium and fluorine, will be shown to be essential for the human system in the near future."

"Is it possible that other elements will also be found to be essential in extremely small amounts?"

"Oh, yes. Much research remains to be done before such determinations can be made. The role of essential minerals is by no means clear or complete. With the advent of new, more sensitive analytical methods, discoveries of new functions can be expected in the near future."

"Well, Professor Carter, get your scientists prepared to research more basic functions being discovered for several minerals, especially for chromium, selenium, zinc, molybdenum and vanadium.

"What do you mean?"

"They should be prepared to study the minerals in such roles as the fine control of DNA synthesis, mechanisms of development, the onset of old age and arteriosclerosis."

"Thank you, but how can you be so sure?"

"That is our job. Out of the over one hundred elements, ninety occur in nature either in a free state or in combination with other elements, right?"

"That is right. We know of one hundred-seven."

"There are seventeen which are artificially produced by humans."

"What are you getting at?"

"All of the ninety naturally occurring elements are present in the human body except eleven."

"Do you know the eleven?"

"Of course. They are actinium, astatine, francium, protactinium, promethium, technetium, helium, neon, argon, krypton and xenon. They are not found in our environment because they are inert. They do not react with anything, so we can't use them."

"Let me see if I've got this straight. Our scientists are telling us that there are fifteen essential minerals we humans need, and you are telling us that there are seventy-nine?"

"Now you are beginning to see the problem. Some of your scientists think that the majority of elements found in the human body may be contaminants from the environment and not the essential components."

"If that is true, the contaminants obviously are non-essential or undesirable elements. And, since the classification of elements is in a state of change, the toxic and essential elements cannot be classified into ridged categories."

"Which means that your scientists really don't know what minerals are good for you, right?"

"I guess you could say that. We are still learning. All metals exert toxic effects when present in excess. For example, even very essential elements like iron, copper and cobalt can be deadly poisons."

"You are right, Carter, but certain toxic metals, so classed by human understanding because of their adverse effects at relatively small doses, are fulfilling essential functions at more minute concentrations. Essential physiological roles for the so called toxic elements like cadmium, arsenic and lead are important to your health."

"Arsenic?"

"Would we lie? Surprise. You need to understand the nutritional roles of arsenic, an element that you have regarded only as poisonous. If you are arsenic-deficient, you will probably exhibite rough or brittle hair, increased osmotic fragility of the some of the cells, and abnormally enlarged spleens containing excessive amounts of iron. Women could exhibit decreased fertility, low birth rates, and retarded growth. Lactating arsenic-deficient women could also die suddenly with myocardial damage. The essentiality of arsenic should of course not detract from the established fact that higher concentrations of this element pose definite health hazards."

"Well, the balance between emphasis upon prevention of deficiencies and measures against toxicity will be difficult to maintain until we know what trace elements are required in the body, what they are needed for, how they get there and what you cells do with them when they arrive."

"The essential ultratrace elements are universally required for your survival."

"Yes, I can see that our understanding of the biological events that link a trace element to its specific vital function is still fragmentary."

"For your experts to understand this, they need to take into consideration the fact that the amplification machinery of the cells - enzymes, carrier proteins, hormones, key structural sites - is involved. So no single scientific investigation pattern will expose what we know right now about these metal ions. Trace elements are essential because they serve as required coenzymes for irreplaceable metal-ion-activated enzymes or metaloenzymes. They will find that at least one-third of all enzymes involves a metal ion as a required participant."

"Scientists know the uses of only a few of the trace elements. But they do know that they are necessary for the work of the bodily compounds of enzymes and hormones."

"It appears to us that the difference with your understanding of what minerals are essential for your good health and what we consider as being essential for our good health are light years apart. Nutrient interrelationships are much more complex than your scientists can imagine, especially among the trace elements. A mineral cannot be left out without affecting at least two other minerals, each of which will then affect two others. Any movement of one mineral will result in the movement of all the other minerals. The extent of effect upon each mineral will depend upon the mineral quantity and the number of enzymes or biochemical reactions the mineral is involved in. This relationship of minerals goes beyond just the minerals extending into and affecting the vitamins, hormones and neurological functions of this body."

"Sounds to me like one would have to be a scientist just to be able to mix the right minerals together, Larry."

"You don't have to be a scientist simply because this is common knowledge to all of the cells of your body. They already know the best elemental relationships."

"Can you expand upon that just a little? I really hadn't thought about mineral compatibility in the body before."

"Two relationships exist among the trace elements, antagonistic and synergistic, which occur at two levels, metabolic and absorptive. Antagonism at the absorptive level is due to inhibited absorption; that is excess intake of a single element can decrease the intestinal absorption of another element. As an example, a high intake of calcium depresses intestinal zinc absorption, while an excess intake of zinc can depress copper absorption."

"And at the metabolic level?"

"Antagonisms at the metabolic level occur when an excess of one element interferes with the metabolic functions of another or contributes to its excretion due to compartmental displacement. This happens with zinc and copper, cadmium and zinc, iron and copper, calcium, magnesium and phosphorus."

"That is how minerals work against each other. Now how do they work together?"

"Carter, we use many different minerals all the time in our work; much the same way you use different tools to work on a machine. And because each mineral has its own ionic or electrical signature, our work goes much better if we have the right minerals available to us at the right time."

"And what if you don't have the right mineral at the time you need it?"

"Just like you with tools, if the right element is not immediately available, we will use the mineral that comes closest to the one we need."

"Doesn't that cause problems?"

"Sometimes. But many times we can get away with it and you will never know the difference until symptoms of some unexplained illness begins to occur. So it is best to make sure that we have a good supply of minerals so that we can select the ones we need to produce the right enzyme or hormone to do that which is necessary at that time."

"What elements work best together?"

"We need all of the elements, but here are some examples of how the synergism between the elements occurs on a metabolic level. For example, we use copper to help us utilize iron. We use magnesium to help us retain potassium in the cells. The synergism between calcium, magnesium and phosphorus is well known to your scientists. But other mineral synergisms include:

Element	Synergistic Minerals
Ca	Mg, P, Cu, Na, K, Se
Mg	Ca, K, Zn, Mn, P, Cr
Na	K, Se, Co, Ca, Fe, Cu, P
K	Na, Mg, Mn, Zn, P, Fe
Cu	Fe, Co, Ca, Na, Se
Zn	K, Mg, Mn, Cr, P
P	Ca, Mg, Na, K, Zn, Fe
Fe	Cu, Mn, K, Na, K, Zn, Fe
Cr	Mg, Zn, K
Mn	K, Zn, Mg, Fe, P
Se	Na, K, Cu, Mn, Fe, Ca

"Wait a minute. There is a third relationship that you should be made aware of. That is where a deficient intake of an element can allow toxic accumulation of another element."

"Can you give me an example?"

"Small amounts of cadmium intake can accumulate to a point of toxicity in the presence of marginal or deficient zinc. And lead toxicity can occur with insufficient calcium or iron

intake, and iron toxicity can develop in the presence of a copper deficiency."

"You do know your elements."

"That is elementary, Carter. A fourth relationship can also be seen when an excessive intake of a single element produces a deficiency of a synergistic element. Excessive zinc intake will contribute to a copper deficiency. Such an imbalance can cause iron to build up in storage tissues. Manganese by interfering with magnesium can result in excessive potassium and sodium accumulation."

"This new insight, suggests that numerous minerals, when in proper balance with one another, may be performing important biochemical functions especially important to age-related health problems."

"We knew we could count on you to see the light."

"Given this body of new data, we should begin to view our daily intake of minerals as performing duel roles; first in the role of preventing known mineral deficiencies; and, second, in optimizing the disease preventing properties of these elements. This information makes it reasonable to believe that it is possible to reduce the incidence of most life-limiting chronic diseases through the adoption of optimal daily nutrient intake levels. The key is insuring that the body always receives an adequate and balanced supply of all minerals that might be of potential benefit to restoring or maintaining our health."

"We couldn't have said it better."

CHAPTER 10

ESSENTIALITY

"Look. All living things are composed of about 99% of twelve common elements from the first twenty of the periodic table. These are the "bulk" or "constituent" elements, whose occurrence in living matter is dictated primarily by their high abundance on the earth's crust, in the oceans, and in the atmosphere."

"However, all organisms, in addition, contain small amounts of heavier elements, which may be somewhat arbitrarily subdivided into trace and ultramicro trace elements. In all, seventy-nine of the ninety naturally occurring elements are in the human body."

"Well, of these, 15 are presently established by our laboratories as essential (iron, iodine, copper, zinc, manganese, cobalt, chromium, molybdenium, nickel, vanadium, selenium, arsenic, fluorine, silicon and lithium,) and at least four others are serious candidates, of essentiality (cadmium, lead, tin and rubidum). Most of the other remaining trace elements are considered nonessential. They are present in the body chiefly as a result of environmental exposure. However, future research could prove that some of these elements have physiological functions as well."

"Then, Carter. Please explain to us what you mean by essentiality."

"The simplest definition of an essential element is that it is an element required for the maintenance of life; its absence results in death or a severe malfunction of the organism."

"Experimentally, this rigorous criterion cannot always be satisfied."

"And this has led to a broader definition of essentiality. An element is considered essential when a deficient intake produces an impairment of function and when restoration of physiological levels of that element prevents or relieves the deficiency."

"So, the organism can neither grow nor complete its life cycle without the element in question?"

"Yes. The element should have a direct influence on the organism and be involved in its metabolism. The effect of the essential element cannot be wholly replaced by any other element."

"So, even if an element might be considered a poison by your experts, if we need it to do our work, it is essential."

"Well, I guess so."

"You see, Carter, a cell passes through several stages as the concentration of an essential nutrient progresses from deficiency to excess. In absolute deficiency, death may result. With limited intake, we may survive but may show marginal insufficiency. However, by increasing the nutrient, a plateau representing optimal function can be reached. Then, as the nutrient is given in excess, first marginal toxicity, then mortal toxicity are attained. While this curve may vary quantitatively for each essential nutrient, the basic pattern holds for virtually all the elements."

"Larrys, dear friends, we are moving as fast as we can towards understanding you and your world. Systematic biological trace element research began with J. Raulin's discovery of the essentiality of zinc for the growth of the common mold *Aspergillus niger* in 1869. Raulin, a pupil of Pasteur and later a professor of chemistry at Lyon, France, demonstrated that *Asp Niger* could grow only if zinc was added to the culture medium, at amounts so small that it could be overlooked easily or considered as a mere contaminant. Raulin demonstrated that the requirement of zinc was absolute, that zinc was irreplaceable and thus essential."

"It is nice to know that you found out that zinc was essential to mold. What about us?"

"Hey, Larrys, this was a new concept. The importance of the concept of essentiality was immediately recognized by the plant physiologists of that period of time."

"What about us."

"While bacteriologists also recognized the importance of trace elements for the growth of microorganisms in the years immediately following Raulin, human nutritionists, with the exception of a few outsiders, seemed to have taken little notice of these developments. Because of this, iron and iodine remained the only two trace elements considered as essential for animals and man until well into the twentieth century."

Well, in the first half of the twentieth century almost all trace element discoveries were made more or less by accident, or in response to emergency situations such as localized outbreaks of unexplained diseases of livestock."

"Good observation. Beginning as late as 1957, trace element research was conducted systematically. This research was dominated by Klaus Schwarz. Experimental methods were devised that enabled researchers to produce specific trace element deficiency states in laboratory animals. This could not have been accomplished prior to the commercial availability of purified amino acids and the development of sensitive and precise analytical techniques, and, in retrospect, was undoubtedly responsible for the delayed development of the field."

"Professor Carter, when did your scientists first know about DNA?"

"In 1953, biologist James Dewey Watson and Francis Crick succeeded in constructing a molecular model of DNA;

they showed it to have a double helix arrangement likened to a spiral staircase. The two intertwined sugar-phosphate chains connected like "steps" with the flat base pairs, adenine-thymine and guanine-cytosine. This model, known as the Watson-Crick model, had a profound impact on biology, opening new avenues of research in genetics and biochemistry."

"Before 1953, humans had no idea that enzymes controlled the DNA chain. So logically, you could not understand how essential trace minerals are to the very blueprint of your entire human body."

"That is correct. For this work Wilkins shared the 1962 Nobel Prize for physiology of medicine with two British scientists, Francis Crick and Maurice Wilkins. Subsequently, while working and teaching at the California Institute of Technology and Harvard University, Watson helped break the genetic code by determining how proteins are synthesized in the cell."

"Okay, back to the discovery of the essentiality of minerals. Please continue to share with us the slow advancement of human comprehension of himself."

"The pioneer in this field, Klaus Schwarz (1977), has emphasized that high toxicity does not preclude biological essentiality."

"Good man."

"Selenium and fluoride are two examples where relatively high toxicity has delayed but not prevented their ultimate recognition as essential ultra-trace elements."

"Good. Now we are getting somewhere."

"There are numerous examples of stimulatory metals. Elements in every group of the periodic table have been found to be stimulatory to growth and survival, including lithium, titanium, gallium, germanium, rubidium, zirconium, antimony, barium, gold, and even mercury. Not only that, but certain relatively toxic elements of compounds when used at low doses can act as therapeutic agents with beneficial effects. Examples are the effect of gold salts on arthritis and platinum complexes on certain cancers."

"The cells of the body do have the ability to substitute elements when the best choice element is not available at the time it is needed. For example, divalent manganese, nickel, cobalt, and zinc may have had similar functions, as illustrated by the observation that these metals can replace the zinc ions in zinc metalloenzymes."

"I didn't know that."

"However, the reconstituted enzyme is usually less efficient whenever a metal other than zinc is bound at the active site, indicating that zinc possesses the optimal properties for that metalloenzyme."

"We use copper to transport electricity from one place to another. How do you use copper."

"In much the same way. We need copper as a part of a coenzyme that is part of an enzyme necessary to build hemoglobin, an important part of red blood cells. About 95% of copper is used in serum as part of ceruloplasmin. Copper is needed by all of the cells of the body, but is highest in the liver where it contributes to energy and detoxification mechanisms. It is also required to absorb, utilize and synthesize hemoglobin, maintain the integrity of the outer covering of the nerves, metabolize vitamin C, and oxidize fatty acids."

"Natural cobalt is often added to hydrogen bombs; upon explosion, many neutrons are liberated, which convert the cobalt to CO_{60}, causing a considerable increase in the total amount of radioactive fallout. How do you use cobalt at the cell level?"

"Cobalt, is an essential part of vitamin B_{12}. It protects against a blood disease called pernicious anemia. Only 0.000002 grams of this vitamin taken each day keeps people

with pernicious anemia healthy, which means even smaller amounts of cobalt are necessary."

"Iodine is needed to form the hormone thyroxine. A lack of iodine in the diet results in goiter, a disease characterized by excessive growth of the thyroid gland."

"Manganese and zinc are required for the normal action of many enzymes. Without these two minerals, certain reactions in the body cells would stop. Manganese is involved in protein, fat and energy metabolism, and required for bone growth and development, and reproduction."

"Do plant cells need the same trace minerals?"

"No. Human beings and all animals need the same trace elements, but plants have different requirements. For example, plants do not need iodine or fluorine."

"Well then, if plant requirements for trace minerals are different than our requirements, how can we be sure we are getting the necessary trace minerals?"

"You can't be sure, because you are not getting all of the essential minerals in your diet. We don't know about all of the other humans, but we do know about you. You see, human beings think they get the required trace elements from their food in a balanced diet, but the information they receive comes from information based on scientific research that simply is not complete."

What do you mean when you say not complete?"

"We believe you can answer that better than we can. Carter, what has happened in trace mineral investigation since the discovery of DNA?"

"Well, let me look at my notes. An essential role in animal nutrition for the toxic metalloid selenium was demonstrated in 1957 by Schwarz & Foltz and subsequently substantiated by others. Within the present decade, investigators have been able to demonstrate that tin, vanadium, silicon and nickel are essential elements."

"That means that eventually all such evidence indicates that present day contaminants may yet be proved to be essential components of life, with the advancement of knowledge and development in analytical techniques, and, all the naturally occurring elements may be found to be present in the human body, thereby proving its microcosmic character."

"That is possible. An increasing number of scientists from a variety of disciplines have become actively interested in trace elements, and a new generation of workers is beginning to make exciting contributions."

"Name some." Larry challenged.

"Lithium-deficient goats exhibited 28% lower weight gains than controls during three months of observation. At the present level of activity, the last remaining essential trace elements will probably be discovered within the next two decades."

"That's too long. It will become necessary to investigate the health effects of all nonessential trace elements, since they all have important controlling functions by virtue of their interaction with other essential trace elements."

"Oh, I didn't think of that. The trace elements would react inside the body in much the same way they would react with each other outside the body, wouldn't they?"

"You simply have no idea of the way these elements are used. There are over 100 binary and five times that many ternary interactions. Of which, we dare say, only a few have been studied by your scientists thus far."

"This is going to be exciting. You will be pleased to know that in recent years the exchange of scientific information between workers in the field has also markedly improved."

"We are interested. Please fill us in."

"In July 1969, trace element researchers from all over the world gathered in Aberdeen Scotland, for the first symposium, TEMA *"Trace Elements in Man and Animals."* Since then TEMA has met every four years. There is also an *International Association of Bioinorganic Scientists* (IABS) founded in 1975. This nonprofit organization publishes the journal *Biological Trace Elements Research* and holds regular conferences on selected topics. The *Society of Environmental Geochemistry and Health* (SEGH) should also be mentioned. Its aim is to provide a unifying forum for research workers in the health, environment, and geochemical sciences."

CHAPTER 11

SOURCE

So, Carter, tell us, how important are minerals to your health?"

"Vitally important? Even more important than vitamins. Ever since we discovered how to overcome scurvy and rickets, we have been taught that it is important to "Take your vitamins." We grew up with vitamins with the suggestive name of "One a Day Multiple Vitamins" to the ones that look like dinosaurs. They came in pills so big we could hardly swallow to the ones we were supposed to chew first. All moms know that vitamins are what keeps her family healthy. But very few know that without the right minerals available to their cells, they cannot assimilate or utilize vitamins even when they are present."

"So, minerals, then are as vitally important as vitamins?"

"No argument there. So what else can you tell me about minerals?"

"Nothing, unless we told you that you need a better source."

"Hold on, Larrys. The source of minerals are limited. I either get them from the plants and animals I eat, or I mine them from the ground."

"You are right on the first part and wrong on the second. You do depend on the food you eat as your main source of minerals, which is both good and bad. It is good if the plants and animals are able to secure for you the minerals you need for our metabolism and healthy growth. It's bad if the plants and/or animals are unsuccessful in their own

metabolism to secure the vital minerals we need. Let's take garden vegetables for an example. They all need various trace minerals for each to grow into healthy specimens. So their roots sink deep into the soil in search of the minerals that are supposed to be there. But for the vegetable to capture the minerals, several things have to exist. The minerals have to be there in the soil. They have to be soluble in water so that the root hairs can suck them up into the plant. The minerals have to be ionic or have an electrical frequency. This is how the roots find the minerals and why the minerals are is important to the health of the plants and eventually, you and us."

"So, I will just simply eat a variety of herbs, fruits and vegetables to secure my trace minerals."

"That is good if they are there. If minerals are sufficiently supplied to the body in proper balance daily, only 25 to 30 instead of 70 grams of protein would be necessary because minerals have a sparing action on vitamins and protein, meaning that less are necessary. Carter, you can stay well by taking minerals, without vitamin supplements, but you will not remain well by taking vitamins without minerals in some form."

"Okay, okay. You have made your point. The earth is a macrocosm, in which all of the active elements are found and my body is a microcosm in which all of the active elements are found."

"You got it. Carter. See it didn't take that long."

"You cells think you are so smart. So tell me where is the best source of liquid ionic trace minerals?"

"The mineral supply is abundant if you know where to look for them. There is a reason for this. Three billion body cells die every minute. In good health or in youth, when mineral supply in high, we are able to replace these cells as fast as they die. But during aging or illness, when the mineral

supply is depleted, the cell growth slows down and reproduction finally stops, resulting in death."

"The person is said to have died of natural causes and/or old age, whereas you believe the cause may have been a mineral deficiency."

"There are many amazing cases of regeneration from adding minerals alone to the diet. Minerals may also be a means of keeping you young."

"Come on, guys. Isn't this going a bit too far?"

"Carter, you do not need to die around seventy, the average age of human death. Look at those great patriarchs who have lived far beyond the one hundred year mark during biblical days before the flood."

"Yes, we read that Adam was over nine hundred years old when he died. Methuselah was almost one thousand years, and Noah was over six hundred when he built the ark. But..."

"Well. Come on Carter. What happened?"

"What do you mean, what happened?"

"What happened to change the earth?"

"You mean the Flood?"

"Of course. The Flood. Why do you think people lived so long before the flood?"

"Because the food they ate had access to all of the essential elements necessary for long life?"

"Bingo. Give that man a super saturated naturally grown carrot from the days when men lived the age of trees!"

"Hey, you just might be right. The Lord told Noah that after the Flood, people would only have the life expectancy of one hundred twenty years. Oh, Larrys, all of you. You never cease to amaze me."

"The flood covered the whole earth. The water came from the sky for forty days and forty nights. It didn't have any minerals in it so the water soluble minerals simply diffused into the water. When the water finally receded, it took many of the liquid ionic trace minerals with it."

"So, if the plants are not able to find the minerals because they were depleted from the soil either by extensive planting of the same crop year after year, or the minerals were washed away by erosion..."

"Or flood."

"... or flood. That would mean we would have to go without or find another source and supplement the minerals in our diet."

"You are quick, Al. When something hits you right square between the eyes, you see it."

"Don't bother me. I'm on to something. If these minerals were washed away, we could logically follow them into the water."

"Hold it. Right there. Tell us all you can about fresh water."

"What is this, a quiz? I am the Professor. I give the quizzes around here."

"Well, Professor. You are about to flunk this course."

"All right, just to please you. Fresh water is water that contains a relatively low concentration of dissolved mineral solids. The quantity of totally dissolved solids varies considerably and depends on a number of factors, including: the total dissolved-solids content of the precipitation contributing to the water body; the nature of the soil and rock through which the water must pass to reach the water body; and human activities (such as the use of sodium chloride or calcium chloride for snow and ice removal) in adjacent areas. Soil and rock are generally the most important influences; in urbanized areas, however, human activities may be equally significant.

"Fresh water usually has a maximum total dissolved-solids content of a few hundred milligrams per liter. In contrast, rainwater generally has less than 50 mg/l (1 mg/l = 1 part per million), and seawater in the open ocean generally contains 35,000 mg/l of total dissolved solids. Brackish waters (those found in estuaries where rivers mix with the ocean) have total dissolved-solids concentrations ranging from 1,000 to 5,000 mg/l. Inland waters having concentration ranges of 2,000 to 10,000 and 10,000 to 30,000 mg/l may be classified as moderately and severely saline waters. The major dissolved substances in fresh water are the cations; (positively charged ions) sodium, calcium, magnesium, potassium, and ferrous iron; and the anions; (negatively charged ions) chloride, bicarbonate, carbonate, and sulfate. Small quantities of nutrients (nitrates and phosphates) are also generally present, along with trace amounts of numerous other elements."

"That is good. We are impressed. Now tell us about seawater."

"Seawater represents approximately 97.2% of the total volume of the world's water and covers more than 70% of the planet's surface. The chemical composition of seawater has been determined throughout geologic time by the erosion of minerals from continental landmasses and the outgassing of volatiles (dissolved gases) from cracks in the ocean floor. Today the ratio of major elements to each other remains nearly constant, regardless of location within the world's oceans. This occurs because the constant influx of minerals into the ocean basins is balanced by a corresponding precipitation of minerals onto the ocean floor. Seawater is a solution of salts; of the various elements combined in these salts, chlorine alone constitutes 55% by weight of all the dissolved matter, and sodium, 31%.

"The absolute amount of salt in seawater, however, is determined by processes, such as precipitation and evaporation, that either add freshwater to or subtract it from the sea. In oceanic areas where precipitation exceeds evaporation, such as in the North Pacific, the salt content, or salinity, of seawater is in the range of 32-34 g/kg, or parts per thousand. In oceanic areas where evaporation exceeds precipitation, such as the Indian Ocean, the salt content may exceed 36 g/kg of seawater.

"In addition to its major chemical constituents, seawater also contains trace amounts of all the other elements of the periodic table. Some of these elements are particularly important, because they form the basis of life in the oceans. These nutrients include such substances as nitrate, phosphate, iron, and manganese. The physical properties of seawater, such as viscosity, density, and conductivity, are determined largely by a combination of temperature and salinity; the biological properties, including pH, oxygen content, and nutrients, are largely determined by the activity of marine flora and fauna."

"Of the two, Carter, fresh water, or seawater, where would you go to secure the greatest quantity of minerals?"

"Seawater, of course. Oh, I get it. You are showing me where I can get my supply of minerals. Larry, we could bottle this stuff and sell it to people who are dying of mineral deficiency. They would buy it right away."

"Oh, what is the use? We will never understand humans."

"Wha ... Did I type something you don't like?"

"What happens to all of the ionic minerals that are washed away from the soil but never make it to the ocean?"

"The liquid ionic trace minerals will all get to the ocean eventually. Won't they?"

"What about the minerals in the mountains and fields of the Wasatch Front, the mountain range in central Utah? When

they are washed away they make it only as far as the Great Salt Lake."

"Yeah. You are right."

"Tell us about the Great Salt Lake."

"The Great Salt Lake, a shallow, saline inland sea, lies in northwestern Utah between the Wasatch Mountains and the Great Salt Lake Desert to the west. Although it receives fresh water from the Bear, Jordan, and Weber rivers, it has no outlet and is one of the world's most saline bodies of water. Table salt, which constitutes three quarters of its mineral salts, has been harvested for many years. All other minerals are found in the lake."

"The minerals in the Great Salt Lake are ten times more concentrated than the ocean. Remove the salt and what do you have? Simply the greatest source of all of the vital essential ionic minerals necessary for good health in both plants and animals!"

"Okay. So we won't bottle the ocean. We will bottle the Great Salt Lake after we remove most of the sodium. Let's see. We can call it, The Elixir of Youth. We could ...

"Carter. Professor Carter. Calm down. It is heating up in here. You don't have to bottle anything."

"Why not? This is a break through in human health."

"You don't have to because somebody is already doing it."

"Oh."

"That bottle of tablets you have been taking every day. You know. The ones that have made your skin young and smooth and your feet soft and supple."

"That's it?"

"Yes. And if you think it is doing wonders you can see in the mirror, just think what we are able to do with those trace minerals on the inside of your body!"

"Wow. To duplicate this natural phenomenon scientists would have to process tons of a variety of herbs, or some how catch the many ionic minerals from the hundreds of thousands of gallons of water rushing down the river. This, of course would be impossible. Think about it. Our scientists can't do it. But the accumulation of all these vital minerals couldn't have been done better, easier or more economically. It has simply been overlooked. Use the Great Salt Lake mineral source and add to it some natural vitamin sources and you have the most potent cell food imaginable."

"We couldn't have said it better."

"I know."

CHAPTER 12

MINERALS

It was Friday morning. I was on my way to the office when I began to feel the swelling up of fluids on both sides of my head. My ears began to pop like I was coming down for a landing in a commercial airplane. By the time I was opening the office door, my head was throbbing. My only salvation was the computer. I had to get to the computer. My eyesight began to blur as my shaking hands fumbled for the key to the door of my private office. I dropped the keys. As I bent over to pick them up, my head nearly exploded.

"All right. I'm almost there," I blurted, as I recaptured my keys from the floor and tried again to focus on the right key. "Back off my optic nerve!" I demanded. "I can't even see the key." Immediately, there was relief. I could see my hands and the keys again. Hey, they obey my demands, I thought. I should have done that earlier. "Get out of my cochlea," I said out loud. "And stay away from my inner ears until I call for you," I scolded as if I was talking to a group of students who were looking out the windows when they should be in their seats. Once again the relief was immediate. I opened the door, sat down to the computer and pressed the power switch. Again I felt the surge of pressure on both sides of my head. "DOWN!" I demanded. It worked. No pain. I purposely slowed my actions. I dusted the screen, the desk, the top of the computer. I straightened the papers on my desk, checked my finger nails, then slowly and deliberately turned to the computer and positioned the headset on my ears. Then I typed, "Do you have something to tell me?"

"Professor Carter, you were watching the ten o'clock news last night. Did you catch what was said about people who are living longer?"

"Wait a minute. How do you know I was watching the news?" I typed.

"We were watching it with you." The response showed up on the screen.

"How can that be? You are inside my body."

"A few of us positioned ourselves in various parts of your primary visual cortex and we are able to see what you see much the same way you watch television, only we cannot switch channels. We see what your eyes are picking up."

"Are you able to hear what I hear?"

"We are able to hear almost everything that happens outside your body but it is muffled. If we want to hear things clearly, a few of us position ourselves at the tympanic membrane, the eardrum and we can hear all."

"I didn't know you had ears."

"We don't. We don't need them. The vibrations are all the same."

"Interesting. So you saw and heard the ten o'clock news last night?"

"Yes. And they were talking about the people who live in a valley in Utah who live twelve to fifteen years longer than the national average."

"Yes. so ..."

"Carter, don't you see? That is what we are talking about; a longer and healthier life for you."

"You want me to move to Cache Valley? They were talking about the people who live in Cache Valley."

"No. It is not necessary to move to Cache Valley. We know why they are living longer."

"Larrys, even our scientists don't know why they are living longer. That is why the federal government is providing a grant to study those people."

"We have already determined how much your scientists know and how fast they are learning, and what they are willing to tell you. And at the rate they are going, you will expire before they publish information you will be able to use. Look, your long life and health is our job."

"Oh, I get it. You are trying to tell me that the minerals in the soil will provide a long and healthy life."

"No. We are saying the lack of the essential minerals in your body make it impossible for us to keep you healthy thus providing you a long life. Professor Carter, the people in Cache Valley who are living twelve to fifteen years longer simply have access to the minerals the rest of the people of the nation are lacking."

"You just might be right, oh Cytotoxic T Cells. You have been right so far."

"Some minerals are available to everybody in the world, but unlike sodium and potassium, which are staple elements of the diet and are present in ample amounts in all food of vegetable and animal origin, certain minerals are additional dietary requirements. Although most are present in the average diet, these minerals may not always be ingested in quantities sufficient to satisfy our metabolic needs, especially during growth, stress, trauma, and blood loss, and in some diseases."

"Well then, let's go through some of these minerals and see how you can help me live longer. The body's requirements for calcium are generally met by eating or drinking dairy products, especially milk. However, it is also found in seafood, green leafy vegetables, almonds, filberts, sesame seeds, asparagus, blackstrap molasses, brewer's yeast, carob, collards, dulse, figs, kelp, oats, prunes, tofu, whey and yogurt. "

"Don't forget The Great Salt Lake. Most calcium (90 percent) is stored in bone, with a constant exchange occurring among blood, tissue, and bone. The intake is balanced by losses in urine and feces."

"And you control the balance of calcium?"

"Yes, by enzymic activity. The blood levels of calcium and its intestinal absorption, deposition, or mobilization from bone are all controlled by a complex interplay of vitamin D, parathyroid hormone, and calcitonin."

"I have always known that I need calcium for strong bones."

"Besides promoting rigidity in bones and teeth, calcium is needed for muscle growth, muscle contraction and for the prevention of muscle cramps. It is also important in the maintenance of regular heart beat and the transmission of nerve impulses. We use calcium in blood clotting and in the protein structuring of RNA and DNA. It is also involved in the activation of several enzymes and in maintaining the integrity of intracellular cement and cellular membranes."

"I suppose that is why during periods of growth, pregnancy, and lactation, calcium intake needs to be supplemented."

"An excellent idea, Carter."

"Thank you for your information on how you use calcium, little Larrys, let's see what you know about phosphorus. I know that phosphorus, exclusively in the form of phosphates, is found in all forms of life."

"Yes. Phosphates are essential to the energy-transfer reactions necessary to sustain life processes. Of major importance to all of the cells of your body is adenosine

triphosphate (ATP), which is involved in nearly every metabolic or photosynthetic reaction."

"ATP is manufactured in the mitochondria isn't it?"

"Yes sir. Reactions that are not spontaneous themselves are driven by the chemical energy released when a high-energy phosphate group is released from ATP. The resultant adenosine diphosphate (ADP) reforms to ATP for further participation in reactions."

"The *tri* in adenosine triphosphate (ATP), means that there are three energy bonds. The *di* in adenosine diphosphate (ADP) stands for two energy bonds. When ATP changes to ADP, energy is released for any number of cellular functions."

"Carter. We are truly amazed with your understanding of our world. A release of energy can be measured even at the cell level. Please continue."

"Phosphates are also important ingredients of bone. The human skeleton contains about 3 pounds of phosphates as calcium phosphate."

"Phosphates also form part of a number of coenzymes and the parts of the nucleic acids that comprise chromosomes."

"Elemental phosphorus is extremely poisonous."

"If you are stupid enough to take it straight, that is, but phosphorus ingested as phosphates in your diet is not toxic at all. A deficiency of phosphorus is rare because it is found in most foods. Significant amounts of phosphorus are contained in asparagus, bran, brewer's yeast, corn, dairy products, eggs, fish, dried fruit, garlic, legumes, nuts, sesame, sunflower and pumpkin seeds, meats, poultry, salmon and whole grain. Again, an overlooked source for phosphorus would be the liquid ionic trace minerals harvested directly from the Great Salt Lake."

"Iodine was first observed in 1811 by Bernard Courtois, a saltpeter manufacturer. In his manufacturing process he used the ashes of various seaweeds washed ashore on the beaches of Normandy and Brittany. While washing these ashes in sulfuric acid he noticed a dark, solid precipitate. The precipitate sublimed upon heating, forming a violet vapor that condensed on cold surfaces as a dark, crystalline solid. Although he suspected the importance of this discovery, Courtois had neither equipment nor funds to carry out the investigation necessary to ascertain its true nature. He therefore asked Charles Bernard Desormes and Nicholas Clement to complete the work, and it was they who announced the discovery of a new element."

"See, there you have it. Humans claim they discovered a new element as if it had never been there. We cells knew about it and have used it all the time."

"In 1813, Sir Humphrey Davy's electrical experiments indicated the substance was unknown to humans. Further proof was supplied by Joseph Gay-Lussac's classic chemical experiments, and it was he who named the element for the color of its vapor."

"The one important function of iodine is associated with the synthesis of thyroxine and the function of the thyroid gland."

"I can see why persons living in coastal regions usually receive an adequate supply of iodine because of the high content in seafood and kelp. But, in geographic regions located far inland, however, a lack of iodine in food is apt to occur, causing goiter. To protect an inland population from goiter, a small amount of iodine is often added by manufacturers of table salt (iodized salt).

"What about iron?"

In the United States adults ingest up to 20 mg of iron daily. Iron is found in eggs, fish, liver, meat, poultry, green leafy vegetables, whole grains, almonds, avocados, beets, blackstrap molasses, brewer's yeast, dates, kelp, lintels, parsley, peaches, pears, dried prunes, pumpkins, raisins, rice, sesame seeds and soybeans."

"Yes, but of that amount, about 0.5 to 1.0 mg is absorbed in healthy humans. The rest is sluffed off unless you are iron deficient, then we could use up to fourfold."

"Iron in food may exist primarily as inorganic, or ferrous iron and a smaller portion as ferric iron. How is it changed from iron in the food to iron in the body?"

"The income of iron is an energy-dependent process that occurs almost entirely in the duodenum. After uptake by the intestinal cell, iron enters an iron pool where it is stored as protein-bound ferric iron or eventually transferred from the cell. The substance in the red blood cells that is largely responsible for its ability to carry oxygen and carbon dioxide is hemoglobin, the material that gives the cells their red color. It is a protein complex comprised of many linked amino acids, and occupies almost the entire volume of a red blood cell. Essential to its structure and function is iron."

"Ah ha, anemia is the loss of the oxygen-carrying capacity of the blood resulting from a deficiency in quantity or quality of red blood cells or the hemoglobin in the blood. Symptoms of anemia include pale skin, weakness, fatigue, and dizziness. Severe anemia may result in difficulty in breathing and heart abnormalities. Iron deficiency, resulting in anemia, can be treated by large amounts of iron in order to gain positive absorption."

"Carter, are all humans this slow to understand these simple health truths?"

"Most humans aren't that concerned about their own health until they begin to develop some of the unhealthy symptoms. That is because you know and do your job so well. What else do you have for us, oh great cells of my body. "

"Magnesium is an essential element in human metabolism and functions in the activities of muscles and nerves, protein synthesis, and many other reactions."

"Prolonged deficiency can cause changes in heart and skeletal muscle. Excessive retention of magnesium can occur in renal disease and results in muscle weakness and hypertension. Magnesium is found in most foods, especially dairy products, meat, and seafood. Other rich food sources include apples, apricots, avocados, bananas, black strap molasses, brewer's yeast, brown rice, figs, garlic, kelp, lima beans, nuts, peaches, sesame seeds, tofu, green leafy vegetables, wheat and whole grains. Naturally, I assume magnesium is found among the liquid ionic trace minerals harvested from the Great Salt Lake."

"You got that right. Carter, we have been talking about several minerals we use in here to do our job of keeping you healthy, but we are intrigued by how you use these same minerals in your outside world. We would like to learn how humans use these very same minerals. Let's make a comparison. You tell us what you humans use the minerals for in your world and we will tell you how we use the minerals in our world."

"It's a deal. Where do we begin?"

"You begin. We will follow."

"Let's begin with copper. Copper was the first metal used by humans and is second only to iron in its utility through the ages. The name is derived from the Latin word cuprum, which means copper. The discovery of the metal dates from prehistoric times, and it is estimated that copper was first used around 5000 BC or even earlier.

"The chemical element copper is a reddish metal at the head of group IB in the periodic table. Its symbol is Cu; atomic number, 29; and atomic weight, 63.546. Copper follows the first transitional series of elements, and its positive ion, displays transitional properties.

"Eleven isotopes of copper are known, two of which are not radioactive and occur with a natural abundance of 69.09% and 30.91%, respectively. Copper melts at 1,083.4 degrees boils at 2,567 degrees centigrade, and has a density of 8.96 at 20 degrees C. The element has a hardness of 3, takes on a bright metallic luster, has a cubic crystal structure, and is malleable, ductile, and a good conductor of heat and electricity, second only to silver in electrical conductivity.

"The outstanding feature of copper is its resistance to chemical attack. Copper is slowly attacked by moist air, and its surface gradually becomes covered with the characteristic green patina that consists of basic sulfate. Copper mixes well with many elements, and more than 1,000 different alloys have been formed, several of which are technologically significant. The presence of the other element or elements can modify the hot or cold machining properties, tensile strength, corrosion fatigue, and wear resistance of the copper; it is also possible to create alloys of pleasing colors."

"That is a good report, Carter. Now, this is what we do with copper. Copper is a trace element essential to your healthy life along with that of many plants and animals, in which it usually occurs as part of the oxidizing enzymes such as ascorbic acid oxidase, tyrosinase, lactase, and monoamine oxidase. These enzymes, which are high-molecular-weight proteins containing 0.05%-0.35% of copper, play an important part in living oxidation and reduction reactions. The metal is tightly bound to ligand sites, containing oxygen, sulfur, or nitrogen atoms on the protein.

"The hereditary deficiency of the protein ceruloplasmin is associated with a pathological increase in the copper content of almost all tissues, particularly the brain and liver. Albinos lack the normal form of the copper-containing enzyme tyrosinase, which participates in the synthesis of the pigment melanin. Copper can be toxic to you in large quantities.

"Copper is required for the formation of aortic elastin and thus is of crucial importance for heart functioning. If you are copper deficient you might exhibit glucose intolerance and abnormalities in cardiac function. Or you may die suddenly with a ruptured heart, caused by thinning of the aortic wall. The copper estimates in typical human diets in the United States furnish less that 2 mg of copper per day, the amount required by adult humans."

"I didn't realize you used copper in so many ways, Larry. It is a good thing that copper is found in almonds, avocados, barley, beans, beet roots, blackstrap molasses, broccoli, dandelion greens, garlic, lentils, liver, mushrooms, nuts, oats, oranges, organ meats, pecans, radishes, raisins, salmon, seafood, soybeans and green leafy vegetables."

"And..."

"And the ocean and The Great Salt Lake." Let's talk about manganese."

"Go for it. Professor."

"The chemical element manganese is a silver gray metal of the transition elements. Its chemical symbol is Mn, its atomic number is 25, and its atomic weight is 54.938. Manganese was first recognized as an element in 1774 by the Swedish chemist Carl W. Scheele and isolated in the same year by his coworker, Johan G. Gahn.

"The Earth's crust contains 850 ppm manganese in chemically bonded form. The name "manganese" is a corrupted form of the Latin word for a form of magnetic stone, magnesia. Extensive deposits of manganese nodules were recently discovered on the floor of the Pacific Ocean and at the bottom of several North American lakes, including the Great Salt Lake.

"Pure manganese is rarely used, as it is a moderately reactive and brittle metal. About 95% of the world's annual production of manganese is used by the iron and steel industry. Manganese is added to iron because it reduces iron oxide to form manganese oxide, which dissolves well in molten slag and is easily separated from the iron. In alloys, manganese increases the durability and corrosion resistance of iron and steel and makes steel more malleable when forged. Manganese steel contains 11-14% manganese and 1-1.5% carbon. This nonmagnetic, tough, durable, and shockproof alloy is used in grinding machinery, wrecking equipment, caterpillar trucks, and mechanical pounding equipment used in heavy-duty construction. The iron manganese alloys, which are used for making other alloys, are ferromanganese (about 80% Mn) and spiegeleisen (15-30% Mn); they contain some carbon and silicon.

"Other important manganese alloys that do not contain iron include the Heusler alloys (18-25% manganese plus copper and aluminum or zinc), which are the strongest nonferrous metals; manganese copper (approximately 75% copper and 25% manganese), which has great electrical resistance; and manganin (about 83% copper, 14% manganese, and 3% nickel), which has a very slight heat-expansion coefficient and an electrical resistance nearly independent of temperature. Alloys very rich in manganese and containing nickel and copper have a high heat-expansion coefficient, however, and are used in the expanding part of bimetal thermostats.

"The most frequently occurring valence of manganese is +2, but +4, +6, and +7 are also common, and +1, +3, and +5 are known. The doubly positive manganese ion has a light pink color in water. Two of the ion's salts, manganese chloride and manganese sulfate, are added to commercial fertilizers. The sulfate is sometimes used for making red enamel, for impregnating wood, and for staining zinc black. Manganese carbonate, yields the pigment manganese white. A number of manganese salts are used in the paint industry to accelerate the hardening of linseed oil and other drying oils.

"When a manganese compound is fused with potassium nitrate, the intensely green potassium manganate is produced. By adding sulfuric acid, the intensely purple potassium permanganate is obtained. Potassium permanganate is used for bleaching and removing color from fabrics that are able to tolerate strong oxidation. In concentrated form such solutions are also used to clear clogged drain pipes.

"The most important manganese compound, pyrolusite or manganese dioxide, is also an oxidizing agent. Pyrolusite is used extensively in the electrodes of dry batteries, where it absorbs liberated hydrogen gas and then chemically bonds it. It is also used as an oxygen source in fireworks and as a chemical catalyst. All other manganese compounds are made from pyrolusite."

"We can see that with human ingenuity, you have found that manganese is very useful in your world in many ways, but not as useful as for your own health. Manganese is essential in trace amounts in human cells, where it activates many of the enzymes involved in metabolic processes. Minute quanities of manganese are needed for protein and fat metabolism, healthy nerves, a healthy immune system and blood sugar regulation. It is used for energy production and is required for normal bone growth and reproduction. Manganese is essential for iron-deficient anemics and is also needed for the utilization of thiamine (B_1) and vitamine E. Manganese works well with the B-complex vitamins to give you an overall feeling of well-being. Manganese deficient humans will exhibit retarded growth, skeletal deformities, ataxia, and convulsions. The defect in the formation of the organic bone matrix, are attributed to dysfunctions of two manganese dependent enzymes.

"The largest quanities of nutritional manganese are found in the Great Salt Lake, the ocean, avocados, nuts seaweed, and whole grains. It is also found in blueberries, eggyolks, legumes, dried peas, pineapples, spinach, and green leafy vegetables.

"Zinc is a metal of major importance in the modern world, Larry. It is widely used as a coating to protect iron and steel from corrosion and as a component of useful alloys. The symbol for zinc is Zn, its atomic number is 30, and its atomic weight is 65.37. The name of the element derives from the German word for the metal, zinc, but the origin is unknown.

"Zinc metal was first produced in India and China during the Middle Ages. The ancient Egyptians used brass, but the alloy was made by smelting copper ore that already contained zinc. The Romans made brass by fusing zinc oxide or carbonate minerals with copper metal. The extraction and production of metallic zinc did not start in Europe until the 1740s.

"Zinc, the 25th most abundant element, is widely distributed in nature, making up between 0.0005% and 0.02% of the Earth's crust.

"Zinc metal normally appears dull gray because of an oxide or basic carbonate coating, but when freshly polished it is bluish white and lustrous. It is moderately hard, brittle at room temperature, and a good conductor of electricity.

"Zinc belongs to group IIB in the periodic table. The metal is a good reducing agent and is used as such in many laboratory applications. Zinc dissolves in aqueous acids or bases, forming hydrogen gas and zinc ion or zincate ion, respectively. Zinc forms compounds only in the +2 oxidation state.

"The two major uses of zinc metal are (1) to coat iron and steel--a process called galvanizing--to prevent corrosion and (2) as a component of several alloys. An additional 5% to 10% of total zinc production goes into dry-cell battery cans and sheet zinc for photoengraving. Zinc protects iron from rusting because it is the stronger reducing agent of the two metals. As long as physical contact is maintained, zinc will be preferentially oxidized; the iron merely acts as an electrical conductor to transfer electrons from zinc to oxygen. The best-known zinc alloy is brass, which is made of copper with 3% to 45% zinc. Die-casting alloys (96% zinc, 4% aluminum, trace magnesium) account for 25% of the zinc produced and are used to make accurately formed metal components by injection molding.

"The most widely used zinc compounds are the oxide, the sulfide, and the chloride. The oxide is used as a reinforcer in rubber tires, a white paint pigment, a ceramic glaze, and an opaque base in cosmetics, salves, and lotions. The sulfide is used as a phosphor in fluorescent lamps and cathode ray tubes and as a white pigment. The chloride is useful as a soldering flux, a dry-cell battery electrolyte, and a wood preservative."

"Of course, Professor Carter, you know that zinc is also an essential element. Zinc deficiency is responsible for Laennec's cirrhosis, a type of cirrhosis that humans formerly thought to be due to alcoholism. Zinc has an accelerated effect on would healing because we need zinc in so many enzymic activities in repair work. It is required by more than 100 different enzymes. It is essential for the maintenance of growth, development, cell division, protein, and DNA synthesis. Marginal zinc deficiency produces a variety of mild or vague symptoms, including inappetence, smell and taste dysfunctions. Major nutritional zinc deficiency causes dwarfism because it retards growth and maturity and produces anemia.

"As you eat each day, we find zinc in fish, legumes, meat, oysters, poultry, seafood, whole grains, brewer's yeast, egg yolks, lamb chops, lima beans, liver, mushrooms, pecans, pumpkin seeds, sardines, seeds, soy lecithin, soybeans and the mineral supplements from the Great Salt Lake."

"You know your minerals, good cells of my body. I know that many of these symptoms have been shown to occur in a surprisingly high percentage of American adults. But, in spite of their central importance, their role in human nutrition are only now beginning to be recognized.

"Let us compare the uses of cobalt. The chemical element cobalt is a hard silver metal with a bluish sheen. Its chemical symbol is Co, its atomic number is 27, and its atomic weight is 58.9332. Cobalt is a transition element with chemical properties like those of iron and nickel.

"Cobalt makes up only 0.001% to 0.002% of the Earth's crust. Never found in its pure form, cobalt is usually bonded to arsenic and sulfur.   Cobalt is also a constituent of many meteorites and is found in the Sun and the atmospheres of stars.

"The name cobalt, derived from the German kobold, a malicious underground goblin or demon, originated in the 16th century, when arsenic-containing cobalt ores were dug up in silver mines in the Harz Mountains.   Believing that the ores contained copper, miners heated them and were injured by the toxic arsenic trioxide vapors that were released.

"Cobalt is a relatively expensive metal used in the manufacture of valuable alloys.   Cobalt-iron alloys have special magnetic properties; for example, Hyperco is used as the nucleus for strong electromagnets.   Alloys of titanium, aluminum, cobalt, and nickel, such as alnico and ticonal, can be made permanently magnetic.   Stellite, an alloy of cobalt, chromium, tungsten, and molybdenum, is very hard and retains its hardness even at high temperatures.   It is used in cutting tools, combustion-engine valves, and parts for gas turbines. Stone saws are sometimes manufactured from cobalt in which very hard particles of tungsten and titanium carbides have been occluded.

"Cobalt Isotopes. Co_{59} is the only naturally-occurring cobalt isotope.   Other isotopes, all of them radioactive, have been artificially produced.   Among these, Co_{60}, which is normally produced by irradiating Co_{59} with neutrons in an atomic reactor, is especially important.

"Natural cobalt is often added to hydrogen bombs; upon explosion, many neutrons are liberated, which convert the cobalt to Co_{60}, causing a considerable increase in the total amount of radioactive fallout. Co_{60} is also used in cancer research and as a source of x-rays for radiation therapy.

"Many coordination compounds of cobalt are intensely colored; several of them are used as dyes, such as Thenard's blue, Fischer's salt, or cobalt yellow, cobalt blue, and cobalt red. The color of some cobalt salts depends on the number of molecules of water of crystallization present. Thus, cobalt(II) chloride varies from dark violet to light red."

"You humans find something good and then you use it for your own destruction. The only real reason for a hydrogen bomb is for the total and complete destruction of a vast number of human bodies. What you don't realize is that cobalt is essential to life, not death. It is especially important that you make it available to us in your nutrition. Carter, you would not exist without cobalt! There is one atom of tightly bound cobalt in the molecule of each vitamin B_{12}. This is important, especially because vitamin B_{12} coenzyme is a compound with a direct cobalt-carbon bond. The corrinoid coenzyme is one of the most efficient biocatalysts, effecting unusual molecular rearrangements in a number of enzymes. While mild cobalt deficiencies, which creates a deficiency of vitamin B_{12}, because it is a cobalt compound, can cause pernicious anemia, it is fatal in the acute form, leading to rapid wasting, anemia, and death."

"Don't get angry, Larrys. We are still learning. That is the purpose of this book."

"But not fast enough. The largest amounts of boron are found in blue cheese, cheese, clams, eggs, herring, kidney, liver, mackerel, milk, seafood, and tofu. Very little, if any, is found in vegetables. But you can always find it in the water from the Great Salt Lake. "

"The next mineral is Molybdenum. It is a silver-white metallic chemical element of the second transition series. Its symbol is Mo; its atomic number is 42, and its atomic weight is 95.94. The name is derived from the Greek molybdos, meaning "lead." In 1778, Karl Scheele of Sweden recognized molybdenite as a distinct ore of a new element; the ore had previously been confused with graphite and lead ore. The metal was first prepared in an impure form by Hjelm in 1782. Molybdenum has a melting point of 2,617 degrees C, a boiling point of 4,612 degrees C, and a density of 10.22 g/cu cm. The metal is very hard but more ductile than the chemically similar element tungsten. It has a high elastic modulus, and of the more readily available metals only tungsten and tantalum have higher melting points.

"Molybdenum is a valuable alloying agent, contributing to the hardenability and toughness of quenched and tempered steels. Almost all high-strength steels contain molybdenum in amounts from 0.25 to 8% by weight. Molybdenum is also used in the "hastelloys," which are nickel-based alloys with heat-resistant and corrosion-resistant properties.

"Molybdenum wire is used for filaments for metal evaporation and as a filament, grid, and screen material for electronic tubes. Other applications of the metal include use as electrodes for electrically heated glass furnaces. Molybdenum sulfide is widely used as a high-temperature lubricant.

"We cells rely on molybdenum because of the many enzymic activities in which we use the element."

"Can you give us an example?"

"Of course. The element is used in the molybdenum-dependent enzyme, xanthine oxidase. A molybdenum deficient body would exhibit a diminished ability to oxidize xanthine to uric acid. But more importantly, an extreme deficiency would cause increased mortality."

"That is interesting, because we humans have never considered molybdenum as being something we need in our diet. Neither molybdenum deficiency nor toxicity presently give cause for concern."

"That is because molybdenum is available in beans, cereal grains, legumes, peas, and dark green leafy vegetables."

"All right, let me tell you what we know about Selenium and how we use it. It is the third member of the halogen group (VIA) of elements of the periodic table, coming after oxygen and sulfur and preceding tellurium. Its chemical symbol is Se, atomic number 34, and atomic weight 78.96. Its name is derived from the Greek selene, meaning Moon. It was discovered in 1817 by Jons Jacob Berzelius in association with tellurium.

"Selenium is a rare element forming only 9 X 10 to the power of -6% of the Earth's crust. Selenium exists in at least three allotropic forms: amorphous selenium is either red in powder form or black in vitreous form; crystalline monoclinic selenium is deep red; and crystalline hexagonal selenium, the most stable form, is a metallic gray. Natural selenium (gray) consists of six stable isotopes and has a melting point of 217 degrees C, a boiling point of 684.9 degrees C, and a specific gravity of 4.79.

"The chemical reactions of selenium resemble those of sulfur and are typically nonmetallic in nature. Selenium reacts directly with many metals. Selenium reacts less readily with oxygen to form the dioxide than does sulfur. Elemental selenium is claimed to be practically nontoxic, but hydrogen selenide and other selenium compounds are extremely toxic, resembling arsenic in their physiological behavior.

"Selenium exhibits both photovoltaic action, whereby light is converted directly into electricity; and photoconductive activity, whereby electrical resistance is decreased with increased light exposure. As a consequence, selenium is used in the production of photocells, exposure meters, and solar cells. Selenium also finds extensive application in rectifiers, a result of its ability to convert alternating electric current to direct current. Selenium behaves as a semiconductor and is being increasingly used in electronic and solid-state devices. Other applications of the element include its use in the glass industry to decolorize glass, as a photographic toner, as an additive in steel production, and in xerographic reproduction."

"Although selenium is rare in your world, it is certainly needed in ours. Long known and feared by humans only as a severe poison, selenium is the functional component of the enzyme glutathine peroxidase. The enzyme assures the maintenance of the structural integrity of liver and other cell membranes by protecting them from the destructive effects of free radicals. Oxygen radicals are formed during lipid

metabolism, but also during exposure of organs and tissues to ionizing radiation, as well as by certain drugs. Selenium is required for the maintenance of fertility, the functioning of the eye, the heart, and the immune system. It also exerts protective effects against certain heavy metals, notably mercury and cadmium. It is also a nutritional cancer prevention agent. An inflammatory, painful condition you call arthritis, is also caused by selenium and/or molybdenum deficiency.

"Depending on the soil content, selenium can be found in meat, brazil nuts, brewer's yeast, broccoli, brown rice, chicken, dairy products, garlic, liver, molasses, onions, salmon, seafood, tourla, tuna, vegetables, wheat germ, and whole grains.

"The chemical element chromium is a lustrous metal of the transition series. Its chemical symbol is Cr, atomic number 24, and atomic weight 51.996. Chromium was discovered in 1798 by N. L. Vauquelin. Its name is derived from the Greek word for color, since most chromium compounds are brightly colored. Chromium does not occur free in nature; in bound form it makes up 0.1-0.3 parts per million of the Earth's crust. The only important chromium ore is chromite. The red color of rubies and the green color of emeralds, serpentine, and chrome mica are caused by chromium.

"The most important use of chromium is in chrome plating, which creates a hard, wear-resistant, attractive surface. Chrome plating can be performed by immersion or by electrolysis. The latter method allows very thin layers to be deposited but uses a good deal of current; the cathode current efficiency is only 10-15 percent.

"Chromium is alloyed with iron to improve its resistance to corrosion, its hardness, and its workability. Other metals, such as vanadium, manganese, tungsten, and molybdenum, are added to these alloys in order to obtain special properties. Genuine stainless steel always contains nickel and chromium. Super corrosion-resistant types of steel, such as those used for furnaces, heat exchangers, and burner heads, contain about 30 percent chromium.

"Important nonferrous (iron-free) chromium alloys include stellite, which contains cobalt and tungsten and is used in cutting, lathing, and milling tools; and nickel-chromium (nichrome), which is used in resistance wire in electrical heaters, irons, and toasters.

"Chromium compounds often have a green color, but yellow, blue, red, and violet compounds are also known. The most important one is chromic oxide, which is used as a pigment (chromic oxide green). Chrome alum forms beautiful violet crystals and is used in the tanning of leather and in textile dyeing. Chromate yellow, one of the most important yellow pigments, is highly toxic because it contains both chromium and lead."

"Traces of chromium are required by certain enzymes for health as part of a glucose tolerance factor. Apart from its role in glucose metabolism, chromium is also needed by some of the enzymes involved in lipid and cholesterol metabolism."

The average American diet is chromium deficient. Researchers estimate that two out of every three Americans are either hypoglycemic, prehypoglycemic, or diabetic."

"We could have told you that. The ability to maintain normal blood sugar levels is jeopopardized by the lack of chromium in your diet and by a diet high in refined white sugar, flour and junk foods. Chromium is found in brewer's yeast, brown rice, cheese, meat, whole grains, mushrooms and potatoes if the chromium is found in the soil, otherwise, it is best to get it from the Great Salt Lake."

"Tin, a solid, rather unreactive metal, in group IVA of the periodic table, has an atomic number of 50 and an atomic weight of 118.69. Its chemical symbol, Sn, is derived from stannum, the Latin word for tin. Tin has ten naturally occurring isotopes; the most abundant is one having a mass of 120 (32.85%). Bronze, an alloy of copper and tin, has been known since 2500-2000 BC. The first inclusion of tin in bronze was probably an accidental result of tin ore being found in copper ore; pure tin was probably obtained at a later date.

"Tin is relatively rare, about 0.001% in the Earth's crust. White tin, the element's familiar allotropic form, is a silvery white, soft, ductile metal that melts at 232 degrees C and boils at 2,270 degrees C. Below 13.2 degrees C (55.8 degrees F), pure metallic tin slowly converts to gray tin, a different crystalline form that is less dense and lacks the metallic properties of white tin. The white form is normally used; gray tin has few, if any, uses.

"When exposed to the atmosphere and moisture, tin forms a protective oxide coating that resists further corrosion. When tin reacts with excess chlorine gas, stannous chloride, $SnCl(2)$, a colorless liquid and electrical conductor, is formed. The reaction of tin with hydroflyoric acid yields stannous fluoride, $SnF(2)$, a white, water-soluble compound that is added to toothpaste to help prevent tooth decay.

"Tin is a major component in many useful alloys. When mixed with tin to form bronze, copper is easier to cast and has superior mechanical properties. Pewter is an alloy of tin hardened with antimony and copper. Tin alloys are also used in solder, bearings, and type metals. Commonly used solders are alloys of tin and lead."

"Tin, by virtue of its existence in the oxidation states and its ability to form complexes with a variety of chemicals, is needed in many enzymes because it acts as an electron transfer catalyst."

"Vanadium is a bright white metallic chemical element of the first series of transition metals. It has the symbol V; its atomic number is 23, and its atomic weight is 50.9414. The element was discovered in 1801 by Andres M. del Rio, but at the time the finding was dismissed as impure chromium. The element was rediscovered in 1830 by Nils G. Sefstrom, who named it in honor of the Scandinavian goddess Vanadis.

"Because the major use of the metal is as an alloying agent for steel, pure vanadium is seldom extracted, and the bulk of the metal is currently made by the reduction of vanadium pentoxide with calcium.

"Natural vanadium consists of two isotopes, V-50 and V-51, the former being slightly radioactive with a half-life of 6 X 10 to the 15th power years. Seven other radioisotopes of the element have been synthesized. The pure metal is soft and ductile, with a melting point of 1,890 degrees C, a boiling point of 3,380 degrees C, and a density of 6.11 g/cu cm. Vanadium is resistant to corrosion by alkali, sulfuric and hydrochloric acids, and salt water, but oxidizes rapidly above about 660 degrees C. Because the metal has good structural strength and a low fission neutron cross-section, it finds extensive application in the nuclear industry. The metal is also used in forming rust-resistant spring and high-speed tool steels; about 80% of the production of vanadium is used to make ferrovanadium or as a steel additive. Vanadium pentoxide is used in ceramics and as a catalyst."

"Vanadium is essential for cellular activity and the formation of bones and teeth. It also inhibits the synthesis of cholesterol. In large doses, the vanadyl sulfate form of vanadium works remarkably like an oral insulin. Sufficient doses of the vanadyl sulfate will completely eliminate diabetes and certain forms of high blood pressure, and once it has done that, the condition does not come back. Vanadium-deficient humans develop higher plasma cholesterol levels. Vanadium acts as a biocatalyst of oxidation of certain substrates. This explains its cholesterol-lowering effect in humans.

"Vanadium is found in fish, vegetable oils, olives, snap beans, dill, meat, radishes, and wholegrains.

"Fluorine is a pale yellow, poisonous, highly corrosive gas. It is the lightest member of the halogens and the most reactive of all elements. Its symbol is F, its atomic weight is 18.99840, and its atomic number is 9. The name fluorine is derived from the mineral fluorspar, which, in turn, is derived from the Latin fluo ("flow"), because until AD 1500 it was used as a flux in metallurgy.

"Fluorine is widely distributed among natural compounds, but its extreme reactivity precludes its presence in elemental form. Although constituting only 0.065 percent of the Earth's crust, fluorine is found in oceans, lakes, rivers, and all other forms of natural water; in the bones, teeth, and blood of all mammals; and in all plants and plant parts. In spite of its ubiquity, as yet no universally acceptable evidence exists that fluorine is a necessary ingredient of living beings.

"Fluorine exists as a diatomic gas. Highly toxic, it has a characteristic pungent odor that can be detected before hazardous concentrations build up. Fluorine boils at-188 degrees C (- 370 degrees F) and its melting point is - 219 degrees C (- 426 degrees F).

"Only one stable isotope of fluorine occurs. The fluorine atom has seven electrons in its outer shell and requires an additional electron for maximum stability. This electron is strongly attracted by the positively charged nucleus because of the small size of the fluorine atom, accounting for the extreme electronegativity of the element. As a result, fluorine has a valance of -1 and forms compounds with all elements except the noble gases helium, neon, and argon. Fluorine salts are called fluorides.

"Fluorine is manufactured by electrolyzing a mixture of potassium fluoride and hydrogen fluoride. It is stored and shipped in containers lined with Teflon or made of a special steel. The latter becomes coated with iron fluoride, thus retarding further reaction.

"In addition to its use in uranium processing, refrigerants, and aerosol propellants, fluorine is used in dentifrices, as a catalyst in producing the dodecylbenzene used to make detergents, and in alkylating olefins used in refining high-octane gasoline, as well as in the production of polyfluorhydrocarbon resins such as Teflon, noted for their nonstick properties and resistance to corrosion.

"Sodium fluoride, NaF, is used as a sterilant, an insecticide, and a water-treatment agent in fluoridating municipal supplies. It is also a paint preservative, it renders enamels opaque, and it is used in dyes and in the primary metal and ceramics industries. Boron trifluoride is a catalyst in the alkylation of benzene for detergent production and in making polymers and copolymers for adhesives.

"Other chemically important compounds of fluorine are antimony trifluoride, an organic chemistry catalyst; sulfur hexafluoride, a gaseous insulator; and several polymers such as vinylidene fluoride. Fluorine compounds are of interest whenever incombustibility or oil and water resistance are important. They are also used in elastomers and in surfactants for the preparation of coatings applied to fiberboard, paper, and cloth."

"Fluorine as fluoride is a requirement to bind calcium in bones. Microamounts of this element are necessary to health. The minute amounts needed of this trace mineral, however, can be obtained in even the poorest diets. The addition of 1.5-2.0 ppm of Fluorine will produce a definite enhancement of longitudinal growth in the first year of post natal life. Fluoride-deficient females will develop diminished fertility and become anemic.

"As to the toxicity of fluoride, fluoride in the water produces a characteristic mottling of the enamel of permanent teeth at concentrations as low as 1.5 ppm.

"Silicon is a dark-colored crystalline semimetal in the same periodic table group as carbon and germanium. The name silicon is derived from the Latin silex or silicis, meaning flint. Its symbol is Si, atomic number 14, and atomic weight 28.0855. In 1811, Joseph Gay-Lussac and Baron Louis Thenard probably prepared impure amorphous silicon by reacting potassium with silicon tetrafluoride. The credit for discovering the element is usually given to Jons Jacob Berzelius, who also prepared amorphous silicon in 1824 by the same method but purified the product by repeated washings that removed fluorosilicates.

"Silicon is present in the Earth's crust to the extent of 25.7% and is the second most abundant element, next to oxygen. The free element silicon is not found in nature, but it occurs either as the oxide silica, in such forms as sand, quartz, and rock crystal, or as silicates in such minerals as granite, asbestos, clay, and mica. Silicon has a melting point of 1,410 degrees C, a boiling point of 2,355 degrees C, a density of 2.33 g/cu cm at 25 degrees C, and a valence of 4. It is a relatively inert element but is attacked by halogens and dilute alkali.

"An important class of silicon-containing compounds is silicones, which are prepared from organosilicon chlorides such as dimethylsilyl chloride. Hydrolysis followed by condensation yields macromolecular structures. The silicon polymers, which range from liquids to hard solids, have useful water-repellent and temperature-resistant properties. Silicone rubbers retain their elasticity at much lower temperatures than ordinary rubber.

"Silicon is prepared commercially by heating silica and carbon in an electric furnace with carbon electrodes. Silicon is an important constituent in several structural materials; in the form of sand and clay it is used to make concrete and brick, and sand is also the principal component of glass. Carborundum (silicon carbide) is one of the most widely used abrasives for cutting and grinding metals."

"Silicon may be the second most abundant element in your world but we need only a "trace" to do what we need in our world. However, if you were silicon-deficient, you might exhibit impaired growth. It would probably show up in bone formations, particularly in the skull. It is necessary for bone and connective tissue formation, for healthy nails, skin, and hair, and for calcium absorption in the early stages of bone formation. It is needed to maintain flexible artreries, and plays a major role in preventing cardiovascular disease. Silicon counteracts, the effects of too much aluminum in the body and therefore, is needed in larger amounts by the elderly.

Boron, calcium, magnesium, manganese and potassium aid in efficient utilization of silicon."

"Nickel is a hard, silvery white metal, familiar for its use in coins but used mainly in alloys with other metals to improve their strength and corrosion resistance. A chemical element, nickel is a member of the transition series and belongs to group VIIIB along with iron, cobalt, palladium, platinum, and five other elements. Its chemical symbol is Ni, atomic number 28, and atomic weight 58.71.

"The Earth's crust contains 0.018% nickel, although the core is believed to be much richer. Meteorites sometimes contain up to 20% nickel. Nickel was mined and used for centuries in its impure form. The first fairly pure sample of nickel was prepared in 1751 by the Swedish chemist Baron Axel F. Cronstedt from an ore German miners called Kupfernickel ("Old Nick's copper").

"Pure nickel is used in electron tubes and in the galvanic (plating) industry, where many objects must be coated with nickel before they can be chrome plated. Most nickel is used in alloys where high resistance to corrosion is important, such as for chemical-reaction vessels and pump parts. Stainless steel, an alloy of iron and chromium, may contain up to 35% nickel. Special nickel alloys include alnico, cunife, and cunico, used as permanent magnets, and nichrome, which is used as electrical heating elements in many household appliances. The U.S. coin known as the "nickel" actually has 75% copper and 25% nickel."

"Inadequate dietary supply of nickel will reduce growth and lower the erythrocyte count and hemoglobin level in blood. Nickel is required for proper iron utilization. However, a lack of nickel also impairs copper and zinc metabolism and lowers the activity of glucose-6-phosphate dehydrogenase and malate dehydrogenase in the liver homoginates."

"Silver, atomic number 47, symbol Ag, is a coinage metal with properties closely resembling copper and gold. Its symbol was derived from the Latin argentum, meaning "white and shining," an apt description of this element. The atomic weight of silver is 107.868, and natural silver consists of two stable isotopes: silver-107 (51.82%) and silver-109 (48.18%). The melting point of the metal is 960.8 degrees C and it boils at 2,210 degrees C.

"The earliest uses of silver are lost in ancient times. Because silver is easily reduced to pure metal from its ores by relatively low heat, and because it is occasionally found free in nature, it probably became the third metal (after gold and copper) that ancient civilizations learned to use. It was well known earlier than 4000 BC.

"Silver is the 68th most abundant element in the Earth's crust and 65th in cosmic abundance.

"Silver is found in minute quantities in seawater.

"Next to gold, silver is the most malleable and ductile metal known. It is harder than gold but softer than copper. This softness limits its use, even for coinage, unless it is alloyed with about 10% copper. When alloyed with 7.5% copper, it is known as sterling silver. As a pure element it can absorb oxygen in the amount of 20 times its own volume at its melting point. It is the best conductor of heat and electricity of any of the metals.

"Historically, the principal use of silver has been for coinage, but its unique properties and the demand for more sophisticated manufacturing methods and product uses have relegated coinage to a minor application. By 1970, 28% of all silver used was for photographic processes, and only 8% for coinage. The remaining 64%, although largely used for industrial uses, was also used for art, jewelry, and miscellaneous purposes.

"Silver's exceedingly high electrical conductance and resistance to oxidation make it valuable in critical electrical contacts, switches, printed circuits, solders, long-lasting batteries, and many forms of electrical and electronic equipment. It is used in bearing alloys for airplanes and diesel engines and recently in some automobiles as well, for the production of mirrors and photochromic lenses, in colloidal form as a catalyst in the manufacture of certain alcohols, as an alloy with cesium in photocells, in the form of silver iodide (AgI) for weather modification by cloud seeding, and in silver-copper alloys for welding.

"Such great quantities of silver are used today that consumption now exceeds production. Its important industrial uses are so great that they overwhelm its use in coins and place several manufacturing uses in jeopardy. Substitutes for silver and its recycling are receiving urgent attention.

"The element exhibits bactericidal properties not fully understood, although these are thought to be a result of its ability to absorb oxygen. Colloidal Silver is used as an antiseptic, germicide, astringent, and caustic and for water sterilization. Prolonged ingestion of even small quantities may cause silver poisoning, called argyria. Symptoms include a blue coloration of lips and gums as silver is deposited there."

"Is that all you can tell us about how you use silver?"

"Oh, I'm sure there are plenty of uses that I've missed, but..."

"What about the medicinal properties of silver?"

"I mentioned that the element exhibits bactericidal properties not fully understood..."

"Not fully understood by humans probably, but totally and completely understood by your immune system. Carter, it is our opinion that your medical profession has not been completely honest with you. They have kept the silver a secret from most of you, so that they could collect more silver in the form of coins from you."

"That is a pretty serious accusation, oh little Larrys."

"Not without reason. Silver has been used by human healers since humans learned how to cough. In ancient Greece

128

and Rome people used silver containers to keep liquids fresh. American pioneers often put a silver dollar in milk to delay its spoiling. Around the turn of the century Colloidal Silver was the medicine for almost everything. Maurice Worthington, M.D. wrote <u>Medicinal Silver Home Remedies</u> in 1928, and the British Medical Journal, 1932 presented an article, Colloidal Silver Preparations of silver in Pharmacy."

"That might be. But our scientists and medical practioners must have advanced beyond silver in their remedies."

"Moved away from, yes, but they did not become more advanced in their remedies unless the securing of silver from you to them could be more advanced. They did that all right."

"Oh, come on, Larry. The medical establishment is not like that."

"Okay, oh great body, please tell us why they would completely abandon Colloidal Silver in the 1930s when it was known to be used as a powerful natural prophylactic and antibiotic? They knew that it was and still is the most usable form of the most effective disease, germ, virus and fungus killer there is."

"Side effects, maybe?"

"Carter, there are no side effects."

"What about silver poisoning called argyria. The symptoms include a blue coloration of lips and gums as silver is deposited there. Nobody wants blue lips."

"That condition was identified a couple of centuries ago when royalty stored food in silver urns, used silver plates , ate with silverware. They had so much silver in their bodies that they became known as bluebloods."

"Really. I didn't know that."

"Here's something else you didn't know. Silver kills all disease causing organisms within six minutes upon contact either inside your body or in the food before it is eaten."

"I should wrap myself in silver foil then."

"You could do worse. Silver fabric is used in burn centers to wrap burns so that germs can't grow in the wound, but you don't have any major wounds that we have been made aware of. We need the silver in here."

"I should buy a bar of silver, grind it up and sprinkle it on my cereal in the morning."

"You couldn't grind it up fine enough for us to use it effectively. It would be best to use Colloidal Silver."

"Why?"

"Because we are in a colloidal environment."

"What is a colloid?"

"A colloid is a substance composed of particles that are extremely small but larger than most molecules. These particles do not actually dissolve but the electrically charged particles remain suspended in liquid because the molecular activity and the ionic effect is stronger than gravity. All of your body's cells exist in a colloidal state. That is our environment."

"Most over the counter medications are in a crystalline state."

"You are telling us? Before any medication can be used, we cells must convert it from a crystalline state to a colloidal state. So naturally, we can more readily use medications already in the colloidal form, as opposed to the crystalline form."

"All other essential elements are used in the enzymic functions of the body, but silver is not an essential element, is it?"

"No. It is not used by any of the enzymes of the body. It is unique in that it works as a death dealing general catalyst against all single celled foreign invaders of our realm but it does not react with any of the healthy cells."

"Sounds like Colloidal Silver could take the place of my immune system ..... Just kidding, Larrys."

"You shouldn't try to kid your immune system, Carter. Your life depends on it. But Colloidal Silver inside the body would make our lives much easier. We wouldn't have to waste time or energy fighting bacteria, germs, viruses or fungi. We would be more efficient in destroying mutant cells, eating dead cells and metabolic garbage. Colds, flu, acne, AIDS, allergies, arthritis, bladder inflammation, candida, cholera, colitis, lupus, lyme disease, malaria, meningitis, pneumonia, ringworm, blood parasites and hundreds of other health concerns would be things that would exist only in your memory."

"Colloidal Silver is that good huh?"

"Better. There are no known side effects, so you don't have to worry about doing harm to the liver, kidneys, organs or any other cell of the body. You can use it externally by applying it directly to cuts, scrapes, open sores, warts, and mosquito bites. It is odorless, tasteless, non-stinging, contains no free radicals, and it is harmless to human cells and enzymes. It is so kind to the body that you can even use it as eyedrops."

THE MIRACLES OF MINERALS

CHAPTER 13

VITAMINS

"Larrys, good biological buddies, we have been talking about the miracles of minerals almost to the exclusion of vitamins. This is very unusual because most health and nutrition books talk about vitamins first and refer to the minerals almost as an afterthought."

"Carter, we agree that vitamins are important in our environment, but without the right minerals in place before the reception of the vitamins, we would not be able to do anything with the vitamins regardless of how potent they are."

Really? I thought you guys were able to manufacture most of the vitamins you need.

We are able to manufacture the nonessential vitamins and others to some extent, but only if we have the correct minerals in place. Vitamins are carbon-containing substances that are required for normal metabolism but the essential vitamins are not synthesized in the body in sufficent quantities to satisfy our needs, so they must be obtained from such outside sources as food, juices or administered orally or intravenously."

"Do you expect me to gather all of the vitamins for you?"

"Mostly, but some exceptions would be vitamin D, which we synthesize in the body to a limited extent, and vitamin B_{12}, which is synthesized by bacterial flora in the intestinal tract."

"So, where do vitamins fit into the functioning of this body?"

"Vitamins and minerals function as "cofactors" in the metabolism of products in the body. Most aspects of bodily metabolism proceed with the aid of specific enzymes but if additional catalysts were not present, for example, the cofactor vitamins and minerals, the reactions would proceed so slowly that they would be ineffective. So, dietary supplements of vitamins and minerals are recommended by us when any of the following conditions are present: unusual diets obviously deficient in vitamins; conditions or diseases causing poor intestinal absorption; and increased tissue requirements that occur in relatively healthy individuals during periods of growth, hard physical work, pregnancy, lactation, and menstruation. Some disorders, including hyperthyroidism, infectious diseases accompanied by fever, and tissue-wasting diseases, also cause increased vitamin and mineral requirements. Also, if you are growing too old too fast or too weak too soon, vitamins and especially minerals should be taken every day."

"Two principal types of multivitamin preparations are available to the public by the medical profession: supplemental, or prophylactic, and therapeutic. Supplemental vitamins contain a range of one-half to one-and-a-half times the RDA requirements except for vitamin D, which should not exceed 400 international units (IU). These multivitamin preparations are designed to help prevent disease and to supplement the diet in cases of unusual stress and other such situations."

"That is all well and good, Carter, but they don't take into consideration the fact that we need many more minerals than the five macro and ten micro minerals previously presented to your nutritionists. Therapeutic multivitamin preparations are prescribed by physicians only for deficiency states and for the nutritional support of severe pathological conditions. Professor Carter, when humans understand that since their life expectancy should be beyond 120 years and if most of them are not reaching that age in good health, they will know they are suffering from malnutrition."

"Well, we do have to understand how to take the vitamins."

"It is not as complicated as some would have you believe. Most of the water-soluble vitamins ingested in excessive amounts are rapidly excreted in the urine and thus rarely cause toxicity."

"What about the fat-soluable vitamins?"

"We store the fat-soluble vitamins in body fat. So they are capable of causing severe toxicity when taken in excessive amounts, as in the case of vitamins A and D."

"How are the vitamins received into your world in my body?"

"Fat-soluble vitamins are absorbed from the small intestine directly into the lymphatic system by the same mechanism we use for the absorption of fat."

"And the water soluble vitamins?"

"Most of the water-soluble vitamin absorption occurs by a passive process. But vitamin B_{12} absorption is facilitated by the elaboration of an intrinsic factor inside the stomach. The intrinsic factor binds vitamin B_{12}, and the complex is carried in the intestinal stream to the ileum, where it binds to a specific receptor site. Here, vitamin B_{12} is disassociated from the complex and absorbed."

"That sounds complicated."

"It is a rough job, but it has to be done."

"If it is all right with you, I am going to list all of the vitamins and some of the specifics of each."

"Please be our guest. We will tell you where they can be found."

FAT-SOLUBLE VITAMINS

Vitamin A (Beta-Carotene)

Vitamin A exists in a variety of forms, including retinol, which is currently considered the most active form. Carotene, a plant pigment present in carrots, for example, can be converted in the human body to vitamin A. Vitamin A is also highly concentrated in fish-liver oils.

Vitamin A has many important functions in the body that relate to membrane integrity, especially of epithelial cells and mucous membranes. It is also essential for bone growth, reproduction, and embryonic development. Vitamin A deficiency has long been known to result in night blindness, in which the ability of the eye to see in dim light is impaired.

Hypervitaminosis A, which results from excessive intake over a long period of time, is most common in children. Symptoms consist of irritability, vomiting, loss of appetite, headache, dry skin, and scaling of skin. Intracranial pressure is increased, and characteristic bony changes are demonstrable on X-ray examination. An extremely high plasma level of vitamin A occurs in this disorder.

"Vitamin A can be found in fish oils, animal livers and green and yellow fruits and vegetables. Foods that contain significant amounts include alfalfa, apricots, asparagus, beets, broccoli, cantaloupe, carrots, dandelion green, fish liver oil, garlic, kale, mustard, papayas, parsley, peaches, red peppers, sweet potatoes, spinach, spirulina, pumpkin and yellow squash, turnip greens, and watercress."

Vitamin D

The active forms of vitamin D are ergocalciferol vitamin D-2 and cholecalciferol vitamin D_3, both of which arise in the body from ingested precursors by exposure of the skin to ultraviolet light. Vitamin D primarily regulates calcium metabolism by determining the movement of calcium from intestines to blood and from blood to bone. It interacts with the parathyroid hormone and calcitonin in controlling calcium levels. In tropical countries, where exposure to sunlight is high, vitamin D deficiency is rare; it is much more common in northern regions. Ultraviolet irradiation of food products, a practice common in some countries, increases their vitamin D content. A deficiency of vitamin D results in failure to absorb calcium and phosphorus, causing faulty formation of bone. In children the syndrome is known as rickets and is manifested by deformities of the rib cage and skull and by bow legs as a consequence of long bones. Adult rickets, or osteomalacia, is characterized by generalized bone calcification and, eventually, gross bone deformities. Symptoms of hypervitaminosis D consist of weakness, fatigue, lassitude, headache, nausea, vomiting, and diarrhea. Urinary symptoms occur when calcium deposits build up in the kidneys.

Fish liver oils, fatty salt-water fish, dairy products fortified with vitamin D, and eggs all contain vitamin D. It is also found in alfalfa, butter, cod liver oil, egg yolk, halibut, liver, milk, oatmeal, salmon, sardines, sweet potatoes, tuna, and vegetable oils. Vitamin D can be converted from the action of the sunlight on the skin.

Vitamin E

Vitamin E is chemically known as alpha tocopherol, the most active of a group of tocopherols; it is present in seed oils, especially wheat-germ oil. Few vitamins have been advocated for more diseases than has vitamin E, including such diverse disorders as coronary artery disease, muscular dystrophy, habitual abortion, and schizophrenia. No persuasive evidence, however, demonstrates that vitamin E has any therapeutic value in these or other diseases. Fortunately it is relatively nontoxic, and few adverse effects from excessive intake have been reported from its use in humans. It is good for the skin.

Vitamin E is found in the following food sources: cold-pressed vegetable oils, whole grains, dark green leafy vegetables, nuts, seeds, and legumes. Significant quantities of this vitamin are also found in dry beans, brown rice, corn meal, eggs, dessicated liver, milk, oatmeal, organ meats, sweet potatoes and wheat germ.

Vitamin K

Vitamin K is essential for synthesis by the liver of several factors necessary for the clotting of blood. Chemically, phylloquinone is the natural plant source of vitamin K, and a synthetic derivative, menadione, is used therapeutically. A wide variety of vegetables, egg yolk, liver, and fish oils contain this vitamin. Deficiency of vitamin K rarely occurs, and its human requirements have not been specified. It is never included in dietary vitamin preparations but is used medically in treating specific deficiencies that occur during anticoagulant therapy, in hemorrhagic disease of the newborn, and in hepato-cellular disease.

WATER-SOLUBLE VITAMINS

With the exception of vitamin C (ascorbic acid), water-soluble vitamins belong mainly to what has been termed the B complex of vitamins. The better-known B vitamins are thiamine (B_1), riboflavin (B_2), nicotinic acid (B_3), pyridoxine (B_6), pantothenic acid, lecithin, choline, inositol, and para-aminobenzoic acid (PABA). Two other members are folic acid and cyanocobalamin (F_{12}). Yeast and liver are natural sources of most of these vitamins.

Thiamine

Thiamine, the first B vitamin to be identified chemically (1926), consists of a complex organic molecule containing a pyrimidine and a thiazole nucleus. In the body it functions as a coenzyme in the form of thiamine pyrophosphate and is important in carbohydrate intermediary metabolism. The symptoms of thiamine deficiency are known as beriberi, a syndrome consisting primarily of peripheral neuritis marked by sensory and motor paralysis of the limbs and, finally, heart failure. People of Asia who acquired beriberi as a result of a diet of mainly polished rice could be cured by adding rice polishings, which are high in thiamine. Today, thiamine deficiency results from liver damage and most often occurs in nutritionally deficient alcoholics.

Food sources of thiamine include dried beans, brown rice, egg yolks, fish, organ meats, nuts, peas, pork, poultry, rice bran, soybeans, wheat germ, asparagus, beans broccoli, brussels sprouts, oatmeal, plumbs, dried prunes, and raisins.

Riboflavin

Riboflavin (B_2) is a complex organic ring structure to which the sugar ribose is joined. In the body riboflavin is conjugated by phosphate to yield riboflavin 5'-phosphate (FMN) and by adenine dinucleotide to yield flavin adenine dinucleotide (FAD), both of which serve as coenzymes for a wide variety of respiratory proteins.

Riboflavin deficiency in humans is characterized by growth failure in children; nerve degradation, particularly of the eyes; sore throat; seborrheic dermatitis of the face and extremities; and anemia. The only established use of riboflavin is in the therapy or prevention of deficiency disease.

Vitamin B_2 is found in the following food products: beans, cheese, eggs, fish, meat, milk, poultry, spinach, asparagus, avocados, broccoli, brussels sprouts, currants and nuts.

Niacin

Two forms of niacin exist: nicotinic acid and nicotinamide. Both are related to the tobacco alkaloid nicotine; in the body they are active as nicotinamide adenine dinucleotide (NAD) and nicotinamide adenine dinucleotide phosphate (NADP) and serve as coenzymes in conjunction with protein in tissue respiration and also as dehydrogenases.

Pellagra, caused by niacin deficiency, is characterized by a cutaneous eruption, at first resembling sunburn because it affects the areas of the body exposed to sunlight. The tongue becomes red and swollen, with excessive salivary secretion, and diarrhea occurs along with nausea and vomiting. Later, central nervous system symptoms appear with headache, dizziness, insomnia, depression, and even overt psychosis with hallucinations and other mental disturbances.

The only established use of niacin is in the treatment of pellagra. Megavitamin doses have been used experimentally in the therapy of schizophrenia. Because nicotinic acid in large doses lowers blood lipids, it has been extensively used in the therapy and prevention of arteriosclerotic vascular disease. Toxicity may occur in the form of liver damage with prolonged large doses.

Niacin and niacinamide are found in beef, broccoli, carrots, cheese, corn flour, eggs, fish, milk, pork, potatoes, tomatoes and whole wheat.

Pyridoxine

Pyridoxine, or vitamin B_6, is a substituted pyridine ring structure that exists in three forms, all of which may be converted in the body to pyridoxal-5-phosphate (PLP), the active coenzyme form. PLP functions in human metabolism in the conversion processes of amino acids, including decarboxylation, transamination, and racemization.

Symptoms of deficiency in humans consist of seborrhea like skin lesions of the face; increased irritability; convulsive seizures, particularly in children; and neuritis resulting in degeneration of peripheral nerves.

All foods contain small amounts of vitamin B_6; however, the following foods have the highest amouints: brewer's yeast, carrots, chicken, eggs, fish, meat, peas, spinach, sunflower seeds, walnuts, and wheat germ.

Pantothenic Acid

Widely distributed in nature, pantothenic acid was first identified in 1933 as a factor necessary to cure certain skin lesions in chicks; its role in human nutrition, however, has not been clearly delineated. Biochemically, pantothenic acid is converted to coenzyme A, which serves a vital role for a variety of reactions involving transfer of 2-carbon fragments (acetyl groups) and which is essential for the production of metabolic products crucial to all living organisms. Pantothenic acid has no specific therapeutic indications but is included in multivitamin preparations.

The following foods contain pantothenic acid: beans, beef, eggs, salt-water fish, mother's milk, pork, fresh vegetables and whole wheat.

Folic Acid

Chemically, folic acid is pteroylglutamic acid, composed of a pterin, para-aminobenzoic acid, and glutamic acid moieties. In the body folic acid is converted to folinic acid (5-formyl-tetrahydrofolic acid), the coenzyme form, which accepts 1-carbon units important in the metabolism of many body compounds. Nucleic acid synthesis cannot take place without the presence of folic acid.

Deficiency in humans results in pernicious anemia and can be produced by antivitamins such as methotrexate, which is used in cancer chemotherapy. Folic acid is present in many common foods, for example, vegetables and liver, but can be destroyed by excessive cooking. Pure folic acid deficiency is relatively rare unless caused by an antivitamin, tropical sprue, or pregnancy. The only therapeutic use of folic acid is in the specific deficiency, although it is included in multivitamin preparations.

The following foods contain significant quantities of folic acid: barley, beans, beef, bran, brewer's yeast, brown rice, cheese, chicken, dates, green leafy vegetables, lamb, lentils, liver, milk, oranges, organ meats, split peas, pork, root vegetables, salmon, tuna, wheat germ and whole grains,

Cyanocobalamin (B_{12})

Vitamin B_{12}, isolated in 1948, is chemically the most complex of all the vitamins, having a corrin nucleus linked to an aminopropanol esterified by a nucleotide and also an atom of cobalt to which is attached a cyanide group. Few vitamins are as important metabolically as B_{12}, because it is involved in many of the synthetic steps required in the manufacture of nucleoproteins and proteins. Almost all organisms need this vitamin but only in very small amounts. Vitamin B_{12} is present mainly in the liver, the kidneys, and the heart. In nature the source is believed to be solely that synthesized by microorganisms.

The ability to absorb this vitamin depends on the production by the stomach of an intrinsic factor, a glycoprotein; cases of B_{12} deficiency often involve patients with defective production of an intrinsic factor. The symptoms of deficiency are identical to the classical syndrome of pernicious anemia: ineffective manufacture of red blood cells; faulty myelin synthesis, leading to a paralyzing neuritis; and a failure to maintain the epithelium of the intestinal tract. Marked anemia and generalized debility eventually develop, which are always fatal unless treated.

Cyanocobalamin has only one established use, which is in treatment of the specific deficiency disease. It is included nevertheless in many multivitamin preparations.

The largest amounts of vitamin B_{12} are found in blue cheese, cheese, clams, eggs, herring, kidney, liver, mackerel, milk and, seafood.

Ascorbic Acid (Vitamin C)

Probably the first deficiency disease to be recognized was scurvy, and as early as 1720 fresh vegetables or fruit were found to cure the disease. James Lind, a physician in the British navy, demonstrated in 1757 that consumption of oranges and lemons could prevent the disease. As a result of his work, the British navy in 1804 made it compulsory to issue a ration of lemons or limes to sailors, who were from then on nicknamed "limeys." Chemically, ascorbic acid is a plant sugar in the acid form, hexuronic acid. In the body ascorbic acid is reduced to dehydroascorbic acid and is involved in oxidation-reduction reactions. Unlike vitamins of the B complex, it does not act as a cofactor.

The symptoms of scurvy result from the fact that ascorbic acid is essential for the formation and maintenance of intercellular ground substance and collagen. The pathology affects mainly bone and blood vessels; teeth loosen because dentin is absorbed and the gums become spongy and bleed easily. In the skin and other tissues hemorrhages occur easily with the slightest trauma.

Vitamin C is used to prevent and treat scurvy as well as a great variety of other disorders, including various dental problems. Although large doses (2 to 8 g daily) have been popularly used to prevent the common cold, many medical authorities believe that the usual daily intake of fresh orange juice provides enough vitamin C for most purposes. Intake of very large amounts for long periods of time can be harmful, although vitamin C has a relatively low toxicity.

Vitamin C is found in green vegetables, berries, and citrus fruits. It is found in asparagus, avocados, broccoli, brussels sprouts, cantaloupe, collards, currants, grapefruit, kale, mustard greens, onions, green peas, sweet peppers, persimmons, radishes, strawberries and tomatoes.

Biotin

Biotin, a complex organic acid containing sulfur, is a coenzyme for several carboxylation reactions involving carbon dioxide fixation. It is synthesized by intestinal bacteria and is widespread in food products. A natural deficiency in humans is unknown, even in individuals on extremely deficient diets.

Biotin is found in cooked egg yolk, salt-water fish, meat, milk, poultry, soybeans, whole grains.

Choline, a simple amino alcohol, is a component of lecithin and of acetylcholine, the latter of which is one of the most important neurotransmitters. Unlike most vitamins, choline can be synthesized in the body, provided that methionine intake is sufficient. It is present in large amounts in egg yolk, milk, and seafood; human deficiency rarely occurs.

The following foods contain a significant amount of choline: egg yolks, legumes, meat, milk, and whole grains

Inositol is actually an isomer of glucose, which is the common sugar of human diets and a component of certain phospholipids. It is vital for hair growth. It helps pervent hardening of the arteries and is important in lecithin formation and fat and cholesterol metabolism.

Inositol is found in fruits, vegetables, whole grains, meats, and milk.

Para-aminobenzoic acid (PABA) deserves brief mention not because it is a human requirement but because it is an obligatory metabolite for most microorganisms and unicellular forms such as protozoa. Sulfonamides, the first successful group of modern chemotherapeutic agents against infections, act as antagonists to para-aminobenzoic acid. In order to survive, most microorganisms need to incorporate para-aminobenzoic acid into the molecule of folic acid. Sulfonamides prevent this, and thus they are inhibitory to the growth of bacteria. They are not harmful in this sense to mammals, because these higher forms cannot synthesize folic acid and obtain it preformed in the diet. No substantive evidence exists demonstrating that para-aminobenzoic acid is a human requirement.

CHAPTER 14

FOOD ADDITIVES

"A food additive is a non-food substance added to food during its processing to preserve it or improve its color, texture, flavor, or value. By legal definition, the class also includes substances that may become components of food indirectly, as a result of the manufacturing and packaging process. A chemical used to make cereal packaging paper, for instance, is considered a food additive if the packaged cereal absorbs it, even in minute quantities."

"We do not understand the reasoning of the human mind. If it is not a food, why ingest it?"

"I know this is hard for you to understand, but humans make money selling food to people who don't have enough. Food additives are put into food for commercial purposes, so more people will buy the food. Some additives are intended as nutritional supplements. Iron, minerals, and vitamins are regularly introduced into foods to compensate for losses during processing or to provide additional nutrients. This is advertised on the outside containers. Iodine may be added to salt, vitamin A to margarine, vitamin D to milk."

"You are not answering us directly. Why add non-food substances to your food?"

"People buy food because they know it will taste good. Flavoring agents make up the largest single class of additives, and include salts, spices, essential oils, and natural and synthetic flavors."

"Not all additives are used to enhance flavor."

"I know. Some additives used to improve texture include emulsifiers, stabilizers, and thickeners. Gums, dextrins, and starches are used to give more substance to soups and desserts. Pectin and gelatin are added to thicken jams and jellies.   Lecithin acts as an emulsifier in dressings and chocolates."

"Some of the additives you ingest we are able to use as foods but others are garbage at best and down right poison to your cells at the worst."

"You must be talking about the additives used to preserve food which are primarily chemical microbial agents, such as the benzoates, propionates, and sorbates that retard spoilage by bacteria, yeasts, and molds. Antioxidants are used to keep fats and oils from spoiling and to prevent discoloration of smoked or canned meats. Ascorbic acid is useful as a means of preventing the discoloration of canned fruits."

"Humans add these non-food additives without any regard for the health of the cells that ultimately have to contend with the chemicals."

"I agree with you Larry. Throughout culinary history, spices and salts have been added to food to preserve and flavor it. However, the wide use of synthetic additives is a 20th-century phenomenon associated with the growth of the food industry. Some of the additives used today are, in the terminology of the Food and Drug Administration, Generally Recognized As Safe (GRAS)."

"What they mean is that it won't kill you, but it might kill us."

"Well, these were used in foods prior to 1958 when amendments to the Food, Drug and Cosmetic Act required that new food additives be tested for safety and there was no recorded evidence of harmful effects. Since 1970, however, the FDA has been reviewing many of the substances on the GRAS list, and a few, such as the artificial sweetener cyclamate, have been banned."

"It's about time."

"Others, such as the sweetener saccharin, have been removed from the list but may still be used. Foods containing them, however, must carry warning labels."

"Check out the new artificial sweetener, aspartame which was approved in 1983 as an additive in foods and soft drinks. And while you are at it, get rid of synthetic food colors, and eliminate some of the dyes. The meat preservatives known as nitrites are very destructive inside your body. You don't need sulfites for use as color preservatives in fresh fruits and vegetables either."

"I know it is hard for you to understand human economy, Larrys, but..."

"We know human economies. The healthier and longer you live the more productive you will be. What is confusing about that?"

"Nothing. You make it sound so simple."

"It is. Forget the non food additives. Concentrate on food supplements. A failure to consume adequate quantities of food energy may lead to loss of weight, wasting of tissues, and eventually starvation. The production of enzymes and hormones is impaired in severe protein, vitamin or mineral deficiency. Just think for a minute what it would be like if all of the proteins, vitamins and minerals were available to us, your cells, throughout your entire life. How healthy would you be? How long would you live? How long would we be able to live? Don't answer that, because you don't know."

THE MIRACLES OF MINERALS

CHAPTER 15

DEFICIENCY DISEASES

"Humans obtain energy from carbohydrates, fat, and protein and also from alcohol."

"That's the alcohol we produce."

"I know that, smart cells. In the majority of societies the most available source of calories is from carbohydrates, and fat and protein are less available. In general, as families or communities become more affluent, the proportion of fat and animal protein in the diet increases."

"Nutritional-deficiency diseases results primarily from a diet that does not have enough of the nutrients that are essential to health or development."

"Another cause is that an individual may not be able to utilize properly the nutrients consumed in the diet."

"Deficiency diseases may result from a person's abnormally high metabolic needs for a nutrient or from some imbalance in the nutrients ingested."

"I suppose certain drugs or medicines may also affect the utilization of nutrients. Symptoms of many of these disorders include severe weight loss."

"The greatest tissue loss can occur in the intestines and liver. But most systems are affected."

"The skin appears dry and pale; the hair is dry and sparse and may fall out. Respiratory rate and heart output are reduced."

"Endocrine disturbances result in amenorrhea in women. Diarrhea frequently occurs in undernourished individuals and can result in death."

"Nutritional deficiency contributes to much of the ill health in developing countries. In these countries the most important forms of malnutrition are protein-calorie malnutrition (PCM)."

"And don't forget endemic goiter and cretinism because of iodine deficiency. But the the major vitamin-deficiency diseases include xerophthalmia, which is due to vitamin A deficiency. It can result in ulceration of the cornea of the eye and increased susceptibility to infection and sometimes blindness. Beriberi, a thiamine, or vitamin B_1 deficiency, is commonly found among rice-eating peoples and alcoholics. Pellagra results from a deficiency in niacin and is associated with persons eating mainly a corn, or maize, diet. A riboflavin, or vitamin B_2 deficiency causes ariboflavinosis, in which there may be cracks of the lips and red, scaly lesions in the genital areas. The macrocytic anemias (involving abnormally large red blood cells) result particularly from folic-acid deficiency during pregnancy and sometimes from B_{12} deficiency. Rickets and osteomalacia (softening of the bones) are due to vitamin D deficiency, and scurvy is due to vitamin C deficiency. Other vitamin deficiencies, such as vitamin K deficiency in the newborn and vitamin B_6 deficiency in those taking certain medications, are much less important and less prevalent.

The specific treatment for each of these deficiency states is usually the medical provision of appropriate doses of the nutrient in question and also an assurance that foods rich in these nutrients are consumed in the diet. This latter approach is also the basis for prevention of these diseases. Some diseases may also be prevented by fortification of commonly eaten foods with nutrients, by various food supplement programs, by increasing local production of nutritious foods, and, in the long run, by better nutritional education.

PERIODIC TABLE

The periodic table is a classification and tabulation of the chemical elements in the order of their atomic numbers that permits systematic explanation and prediction of many of the elements' chemical and physical properties.

ARRANGEMENT OF THE PERIODIC TABLE

The periodic table begins with Hydrogen, an anomalous element, is placed by itself at the beginning of the chart. The elements that follow are arranged horizontally until an element is reached that has the properties of one in the previous period. This is placed below the analog, and a new horizontal period is begun.

The chart so designed can be read either horizontally or vertically. If horizontally, the elements are arranged in a series not only by atomic weight, but also by valence. Beginning with the monovalent alkali metals the positive valence increases to three. Carbon, with its nonpolar valence of four, occupies a central position, followed by nitrogen, oxygen, and fluorine, with valences of -3, -2, and -1, respectively.

Originally there were seven vertical columns below each element in the first period, designated by the Roman numerals I to VII. Further down the table appeared the so-called transition elements iron, cobalt, and nickel. Because the properties of these transition elements set them apart, another column, VIII, was designated for them.

When the table is read vertically, each column comprises a family of elements having similar properties. In this form the table was able to meet the needs of inorganic chemists for the organization of what had previously been a mass of uncoordinated facts. Even though the table as an empirical construction fit the observed facts very well, however, no theoretical reasons for its existence could be given.

The first serious challenge to the neat organization occurred in 1894, when argon was discovered. No similar unreactive gases were then new vertical column, designated the zero column, to the table. Since the gas formed no compounds, it had no valence and so could take its place before the elements of column I. This, of course, implied that other similar inert gases must also exist. With the table as a guide, the other members of the inert-gas family, helium, neon, krypton, and xenon, were quickly found (1895-98).

Francis William Aston showed by means of his mass spectrograph that most elements are mixtures of isotopes. The atomic weights determined by chemical analysis, then, are actually the average of the atomic weights of all the isotopes with the same atomic number. In the case of the anomalously placed elements, atomic weight did not put each element in its proper position as indicated by its atomic number.

As the structure of the atom became clearer, so did the theoretical explanation for the periodic table. Atomic structure was based on the picture proposed by Niels Bohr in 1913. The atomic number was identified with the number of protons--positively charged particles--present in the nucleus of each atom. Balancing this was an equal number of negatively charged electrons orbiting the nucleus in a series of shells designated by the letters K, L, M, and so on. The innermost shell, K, held either one electron, corresponding to hydrogen, or two, corresponding to the inert gas helium. When the K shell was complete, a new shell, L, began to form, building up the next eight elements to the next inert gas, neon, atomic number 10. Thus the electron configuration of the inert gases represented a stable situation that the other elements tended to approach by gain or loss of electrons in chemical reactions. The periodicity of the table was due to the repeating trend toward formation of the stable configuration, and the outer shells could contain 18 or even 32 electrons.

The idea of a regularly increasing number of electrons as the atomic number increased implied that each shell was built up until it was complete before the next shell could be started. This idea could be modified to account for the rare earth elements, which showed an increasing number of electrons in regular order from lanthanum to lutecium but relatively little difference in chemical properties. It is now assumed that before the outermost shell is complete, a new shell somehow begins to form and becomes, in turn, the outermost shell. Meanwhile, the incomplete shell continues to be filled, while the chemical properties determined by the outer shell remain very similar.

ELEMENTS OF THE EARTH
AND THE HUMAN BODY

RADIOACTIVITY

The final vindication of the periodic table came from the study of radioactive elements, which led to the creation of the transuranium elements. Almost as soon as radioactive elements were discovered it was recognized that they decayed at definite rates, giving rise to new elements while emitting rays of three kinds--alpha, beta, and gamma. The gamma rays were soon identified as X rays that do not change the nature of the element concerned. The alpha rays, however, were found to be helium ions with an atomic weight of four and a double negative charge, while the beta rays were electrons whose slight mass did not alter the atomic weight of the elements from which they came.

The loss of these particles from the nucleus altered the atomic number of the element, thus producing a new element. In 1911 and 1913, Soddy showed that loss of an alpha particle moved an element two places to the left in the table, while loss of an electron moved it one place to the right. A decay series of elements is formed by a continued chain of such transformations. Three such series were recognized that started from isotopes of uranium, actinium, and thorium. A plutonium series was later recognized. Obviously a number of isotopes could be formed, and in most cases the end product was a nonradioactive lead isotope. Had the large number of isotopes involved in these events been discovered early they would have been inexplicable, but the concept of atomic numbers made it possible to understand what had happened.

ARTIFICIAL TRANSMUTATION

Once the idea of the interconversion of elements had been accepted, it became apparent that artificial changes might be produced if some sort of charged particle could be introduced into an atomic nucleus. Elements so produced could be expected to be too unstable to be found in nature, since they would decay too rapidly. In the 1930s the Joliot-Curies actually produced artificial transmutations by bombarding metal targets with alpha rays. The cyclotron, developed by Ernest Lawrence, supplied a much more powerful source of particles with which to bombard targets of various elements and permitted Emilio Segre to find the missing element 43, the first artificially produced element. It was named technetium from the Greek word for "artificial." Artificial production of elements completed the periodic table with the creation of promethium, element 61; astatine, element 85; and francium, element 87. All these elements were radioactive and decayed rapidly, which explained why they had not been found by ordinary chemical methods. All fit exactly into their places in the table.

Much more exciting to chemists was the possibility of creating new elements heavier than uranium. In 1940, Edwin M. McMillan was able to produce element 93, which he called neptunium, the first element beyond uranium, just as Neptune was the first planet beyond Uranus. At this point the work on the production of new elements apparently stopped, but it actually continued very actively in secret because the research was connected with the manufacture of the atomic bomb. Glenn Seaborg, McMillan's colleague, continued the latter's work, and large quantities of element 94, plutonium, were synthesized. The results of all this work were finally published in 1946, and open work on the transuranium elements continued actively. Elements as high as 105 have been prepared. It was fitting that element 101 was named mendelevium in honor of the discoverer of the periodic table.

ACTINIDE SERIES

The actinide elements are the 14 chemical elements that follow actinium in Group IIIB of the Periodic Table.

Because of some chemical similarities, actinium is usually included in the series. All of the actinides are radioactive, because their nuclei are so large that they are unstable and release great amounts of energy when they undergo spontaneous fission. Most of the actinides are not found in nature but are artificially produced in the laboratory.

ACTINIDES FOUND IN NATURE

Two of the actinides have isotopes with such a long half-life that they have not completely decayed since the Earth was formed. One isotope of thorium, Th-232, has a half-life of 14 billion years and has an abundance of 12 parts per million in the Earth's crust. It is a principal constituent of some minerals, notably thorite and monazite (a mixed rare-earth and thorium phosphate).

Three isotopes of uranium are found in nature. Their isotopic abundances and half-lives are U-234, 0.006%, 230,000 years; U-235, 0.72%, 696 million years; and U-238, 99.27%, 4.51 billion years. Some laboratory-producd isotopes of uranium also have long half-lives. The overall abundance of uranium in the Earth's crust is about 4 parts per million, and it is concentrated in many minerals, principally pitchblende, autunite, torbernite, and carnotite. Deposits of uranium minerals large enough to be profitably mined are found principally in parts of Africa and in Canada, the Soviet Union, and the southwestern United States. Actinium and protactinium, as well as some isotopes of thorium and uranium, are found in nature as decay products of Th-232, U-235, or U-238. All of the heavier actinide elements, the transuranium elements, as well as some isotopes of the lighter actinides, have been synthesized since 1940. Small amounts of neptunium-239 and plutonium-239 have been found in uranium ores; they are produced by the absorption of neutrons generated by the spontaneous fission of U-238.

LANTHANIDE SERIES

The lanthanide series is the group of chemical elements that follow lanthanum in the periodic table. Their distinguishing feature is that they fill the 4f electronic subshell. Although only the elements cerium (atomic number 58) through lutetium (71) are lanthanide elements in principle, most chemists include yttrium (39) and lanthanum (57) in this group because they have similar physical and chemical properties. They are also called the inner transition elements (because the 4f electron density is relatively close to the nucleus) and the rare earths (because they were originally isolated as oxides, or "earths," and were originally discovered in rare minerals). In comparison with other elements, they are not really rare. Lanthanide elements are found in many minerals, principally in monazite, which is predominately phosphates of cerium, thorium, neodymium, and lanthanum. Lanthanum itself was so named because it is difficult to isolate (the Greek lanthanein means "to lurk unseen"). In igneous rocks on the Earth's surface, cerium is the most abundant lanthanide, but even thulium, which is much less abundant, is found in higher concentration than the elements arsenic, mercury, and silver. The lanthanides, however, are found together in nature and are very difficult to separate from each other because they are chemically similar.

One lanthanide, promethium, has only radioactive isotopes with short half-lives, and its presence in nature has only recently been detected in exceedingly small amounts. Many incorrect claims to the discovery of element 61 were made between 1924 and 1938. It was not until 1947 that scientists announced that this element could be separated from the products of nuclear fission of uranium in a reactor.

In their elemental form, the lanthanides are silvery metals with high melting points. They tarnish slowly in air, except for samarium, europium, and ytterbium, which are much more reactive toward oxygen or moisture. The metals are prepared from fluorides or oxides by treatment with strongly reducing metals like calcium, or from molten chloride or fluoride salts by electrolysis at high temperatures. The lanthanides are typically isolated as a group by precipitating their insoluble hydroxides, oxalates, or phosphates. Until 1945, tedious, repetitive procedures such as fractional crystallization were required to separate these elements from one another. A much more effective separation technique, ion-exchange chromatography, has been used since 1945.

Until recently the only commercial use of the rare earths was as misch metal, an alloy consisting principally of cerium, lanthanum, and neodymium, which is pyrophoric (catching fire in air) when finely divided and is used to make cigarette-lighter flints. Commercial production of the rare earths is now growing by approximately 20% each year. They are used as alloying materials in metallurgy (to remove sulfur and oxygen) and to make strong permanent magnets such as from $SmCo(5)$. Other modern uses are as magnetic oxides such as yttrium iron garnet; aw phosphors in television screens; aw catalysts that decompose auto air pollutants; and as compounds that store hydrogen effectively.

CARBONATE MINERALS

Carbonate minerals are those having the carbonate ion $CO(3)(=)$ as a major component. This ion reacts readily with acid to produce carbon dioxide and water; therefore, the carbonate minerals are generally characterized by their solubility in acids, often with effervescence. The carbonates are further grouped into five subclasses: (1) anhydrous normal carbonates, (2) hydrated normal carbonates, (3) acid carbonates (bicarbonates), (4) carbonates with hydroxyl (OH) or a halogen, and (5) compound carbonates with other anions such as sulfate or phosphate.

All the more common carbonate minerals belong to class 1. However, some minerals in other classes, although rare in nature, may occur in localized concentrations sufficient to be exploited as ore deposits or to have other uses.

The class 1 carbonates are grouped into three structural types. The calcite group consists of the rhombohedral (hexagonal system) carbonates calcite, magnesite, siderite, rhodochrosite, smithsonite, and several rarer members. The dolomite group, structurally similar to calcite, includes the double carbonates dolomite and ankerite as important members. The aragonite group consists of the orthorhombic carbonates of larger radius cations and includes strontianite, cerussite, witherite, and argonite, the high-pressure polymorph of calcite. A few, rare class 1 carbonates do not belong to the three major structural groups, among them vaterite (a third natural polymorph of calcite and rutherfordine. Calcite and dolomite are by far the most common of the carbonate minerals and are among the most common minerals of any sort. Aragonite is abundant in modern marine sediments. The other class 1 carbonates are found in sedimentary or hydrothermal deposits and are often important sources of their metals.

Most other carbonates decompose at high temperatures; hence their occurrences are restricted to sedimentary or low-temperature hydrothermal deposits. The only class 2 mineral of note is natron, commonly called washing soda. It and the principal class 3 mineral, trona, are both water soluble and consequently are found only in arid regions. However, they sometimes occur in large evaporite deposits in closed desert basins, and trona is mined as a source of sodium.

Class 4 carbonates include the copper ores malachite and azurite, which, because of their aesthetic appeal, are prized by mineral collectors and frequently used for ornamental stone. This class also includes rare-earth carbonates, principally bastnaesite. Although this mineral occurs only in rare igneous carbonatites, it is one of the major ores of lanthanum and rare-earth elements.

157

PERIODIC

1A								
1 H Hydrogen	**2A**							
3 Li Lithium	**4 Be** Beryllium							
11 Na Sodium	**12 Mg** Magnesium	**3B**	**4B**	**5B**	**6B**	**7B**	**8B** ------------	
19 K Potassium	**20 Ca** Calcium	**21 Sc** Scandium	**22 Ti** Titanium	**23 V** Vanadium	**24 Cr** Chromium	**25 Mn** Manganese	**26 Fe** Iron	**27 Co** Cobalt
37 Rb Rubidium	**38 Sr** Strontium	**39 Y** Yittrium	**40 Zr** Zirconium	**41 Nb** Niobium	**42 Mo** Molybdenum	**43 Tc** Technetium	**44 Ru** Ruthenium	**45 Rh** Rhodium
55 Cs Cesium	**56 Ba** Barium		**72 Hf** Hafnium	**73 Ta** Tantalum	**74 W** Tungsten	**75 Re** Rhenium	**76 Os** Osmium	**77 Ir** Iridium
87 Fr Francium	**88 Ra** Radium		**104** Element 104	**105** Element 105	**106** Element 106	**107** Element 107	**108** Element 108	**109** Element 109

57 La Lanthanum	**58 Ce** Cerium	**59 Pr** Praseodymium	**60 Nd** Neodymium	**61 Pm** Promethium	**62 Sm** Samarium	**63 Eu** Europium
89 Ac Actinium	**90 Th** Thorium	**91 Pa** Protactinium	**92 U** Uranium	**93 Np** Neptunium	**94 Pu** Plutonium	**95 Am** Americium

TABLE

8A

| | | | | | | 2 He Helium |

| 3A | 4A | 5A | 6A | 7A | |

| 5 B Boron | 6 C Carbon | 7 D Nitrogen | 8 O Oxygen | 9 F Fluorine | 10 Ne Neon |
| 13 Al Aluminum | 14 Si Silicon | 15 P Phosphorus | 16 S Sulfur | 17 Cl Chlorine | 18 Ar Argon |

| 1B | 2B |

28 Ni Nickel	29 Cu Copper	30 Zn Zinc	31 Ga Gallium	32 Ge Germanium	33 As Arsenic	34 Se Selenium	35 Br Bromine	36 Kr Krypton
46 Pd Palladium	47 Ag Silver	48 Cd Cadmium	49 In Idium	50 Sn Tin	51 Sb Antimony	52 Te Tellurium	53 I Iodine	54 Xe Xenon
78 Pt Platinum	79 Au Gold	80 Hg Mercury	81 Ti Thallium	82 Pb Lead	83 Bi Bismuth	84 Po Polonium	85 At Astatine	86 Rn Radon

| 64 Gd Gadolinium | 65 Tb Terbium | 66 Dy Dysprosium | 67 Ho Holmium | 68 Er Erbium | 69 Tm Thulium | 70 Yb Ytterbium | 71 Lu Lutetium |
| 96 Cm Curium | 97 Bk Berkelium | 98 Cf Californium | 99 Es Einsteinium | 100 Fm Fermium | 101 Md Mendelevium | 102 No Nobelium | 103 Lr Lawrencium |

ARSENIC

Arsenic is a metallic chemical element. Its symbol is As, its atomic number 33, and its atomic weight 74.9216. The Earth's crust contains relatively little arsenic, only about 5.5 parts per million. Arsenic occurs in numerous minerals, in particular realgar, orpiment, and arsenopyrite. Arsenic and some arsenic compounds have been known for a long time. Aristotle thought that arsenic was a kind of sulfur. In about 1250, Albertus Magnus became the first to describe a method of manufacturing arsenic. Since then the method has scarcely changed: the mineral arsenopyrite is heated and decomposes with the liberation of arsenic gas. The gas can be condensed on a cold surface.

Arsenic exists in three allotropic modifications: the yellow (represented by Greek lower-case letter alpha); the black (represented by Greek lower-case letter beta); and the metallic, or gray (represented by Greek lower-case letter gamma). Normally arsenic is found in its metallic form, which is the most stable and at normal pressure does not melt but sublimes at about 615 deg C. It forms alloys with other metals. The alpha and beta modifications have no metallic properties. Arsenic is fairly reactive. Above 400 deg C it burns with a bluish flame, forming arsenic trioxide. This compound is known as white arsenic and is used as a rat poison.

Arsenic was used in Aristotle's time to harden copper. Orpiment and realgar have long been used as depilatories in the leather industry. When orpiment is rubbed on silver, it gives the surface a golden color. Orpiment thus appears to have one of the properties attributed to the philosophers' stone, and it was therefore an important material for alchemists.

The toxic quality of arsenic also has been known since ancient times. In the human body it accumulates in the nails and the hair, where it can be detected--even in the bodies of persons long dead--by the Marsh test. The acute symptoms are diarrhea and cramps. In cases of chronic poisoning, anemia and paralysis may appear. If there is prolonged contact with the skin, malignant skin tumors can develop. BAL (British Anti-Lewisite) was developed as an antidote against the arsenic-containing war gas Lewisite, but it also proved useful in treating common arsenic poisoning. In medicine, 4-aminobenzene arsenic and 4-hydroxybenzene arsenic compounds are used in certain infections. The best known is

Salvarsan, an antisyphilis drug. Commercially arsenic is added to lead to harden it and is used in the production of herbicides and pesticides.

In the mid 70s, Schwartz directed his attention to the study of the nutritional roles of arsenic, an element that until then had always been regarded only as poisonous. Arsenic-deficient rats exhibited rough fur, increased osmotic fragility of the erythocytes, and abnormally enlarged spleens containing excessive amounts of iron. Arsenic-deficient goats and pigs showed decreased fertility, low birth rates, and retarded growth. Lactating arsenic-deficient goats were also observed to die suddenly with myocardial damage. The discovery of the essentiality of arsenic and the possible essentiality of lead and cadmium should of course not detract from the established fact that higher concentrations of these elements pose definite health hazards.

BARIUM

Barium is a chemical element--a silvery, soft metal--and it is the fifth of the alkaline earth menals forming Group II in the periodic table. Its symbol is Ba; its atomic number is 56; and its atomic weight is 137.34. The density of barium is 3.75 g/cu cm at 20 deg C; its melting point is approximately 725 deg C, and its boiling point is approximately 1,640 deg C.

The name barium is derived from the Greek barus, meaning "heavy."

Barium is widely distributed in nature. The principal ore is barite (barium sulfate), also called heavy spar. The presence of barium oxide in barite was discovered (1779) by K. W. Scheele, and the metal was first isolated (1808) by Sir Humphry Davy.

Pure barium oxidizes readily, a property that makes it useful as a "getter" for removing oxygen from vacuum tubes.

Useful alloys of barium and aluminum or magnesium are made by reacting these metals with barium oxide.

Barium is highly electropositive and very reactive. It readily forms the barium ion, which has a double-positive charge and behaves as a typical divalent ion and can be used to precipitate larger anions. Barium hydroxide is soluble in water and is a strong base.

Barium oxide, BaO, is used as a laboratory source of small amounts of peroxide. The oxidation of BaO in air produces barium peroxide, which, reacting with diluted sulfuric acid, yields hydrogen peroxide.

Barium carbonate is used as a raw material for other barium compounds, as an ingredient in optical glass and fine glassware, and in the preparation of ceramic permanent magnets used in loudspeakers.

BERYLLIUM

is a chemical element, one of the alkaline-earth metals in Group IIA of the periodic table. Its symbol is Be, its atomic number 4, and its atomic weight 9.0122. A steel-gray metal, its properties are similar to those of aluminum and magnesium, except that its melting point, about 1,278 deg C, is high for a light metal.

Chemically, beryllium differs markedly from the other alkaline-earth metals in that it forms compounds that are more covalent than ionic.

Beryllium is a rare element: its concentration in the Earth's crust is approximately 6 ppm, and no rich deposits of it exist. It is produced from the mineral beryl. (Emeralds and aquamarines are forms of beryl.)

The element was discovered, in its oxide form, by the French chemist Louis Nicolas Vauquelin in 1798. The metal was first prepared in 1828 by Friedrich Wohler and Antoine Bussy, working independently.

In metallurgy, the specific applications of beryllium are based on its high ratio of strength to weight--it is lighter and yet much stronger than aluminum--and on its high melting point. In addition, it forms a strong oxide layer on its surface, which gives it a high corrosion resistance, as high as that of aluminum.

ELEMENTS OF THE EARTH
AND THE HUMAN BODY

The addition of traces of beryllium to alloys can greatly increase their corrosion resistance. But the cost of beryllium, which is about 200 times that of aluminum, restricts its applications to a few special ones, such as in computer components, gyroscopes, and space technology.

The most important beryllium alloy is beryllium copper (up to 4% Be), which is obtained by fusing beryllium oxide with copper, with carbon as a reducing agent. Beryllium copper is used in corrosion-resistant springs, electrical contacts--beryllium is a little less than half as conductive as copper--and, because of its hardness, in spark-proof tools. (Spark-proof hammers and wrenches are used in work with highly flammable materials.)

Beryllium is important in nuclear-reactor technology because it is an excellent neutron reflector and moderator. For this reason, and because of its strength and great resistance to heat, beryllium is employed as a cladding material for nuclear fuel elements.

Beryllium, when bombarded with alpha radiation, emits a large number of neutrons; this was how the neutron was discovered in 1932.

The most important beryllium compound is beryllium oxide, BeO. It is used as a base material in ceramics and in special types of glass; in fluorescent tubes; and in nuclear reactors.

Beryllium and its compounds are extremely toxic. Inhalation of dust particles or vapors containing beryllium may cause berylliosis, an inflammation of the lungs.

BISMUTH

The chemical element bismuth is a soft, brittle, highly lustrous metal belonging to the same group in the periodic table as arsenic. Its symbol is Bi; its atomic number is 83; its atomic weight is 208.9806.

The discoverer of the element is unknown, as is the origin of its name. No record exists of its use in ancient times, but Europeans had become aware of its existence by the Middle Ages.

The average abundance of bismuth in the Earth's crust is about 0.00002%. It is most commonly found as an oxide, sulfide, or carbonate in silver, lead, zinc, and tin mineral deposits. The metal is a by-product of the smelting of these ores.

Bismuth metal has a melting point of 271 deg C (520 deg F) and a boiling point of 1,560 deg C (2,840 deg F). On freezing, molten bismuth expands 3.3% by volume, a property shared by only one other element, gallium.

Bismuth forms compounds in the +3 and +5 oxidation states; the +3 state is the more stable of the two. The metal dissolves in nitric acid to form bismuth nitrate, which on controlled hydrolysis produces bismuth subnitrate. Other mixed oxide salts of bismuth are similarly named.

The very low toxicity of ordinary bismuth salts permits their use in the cosmetic and pharmaceutical industries. An important new application is the use of the complex salt bismuth phosphomolybdate as an industrial catalyst in the synthesis of acrylonitrile, an intermediate product in the manufacture of acrylic fibers, ABS plastic, and Lucite paints.

BORON

Boron is a metalloid chemical element with properties intermediate between those of carbon and aluminum. Its chemical symbol is B, atomic number 5, and atomic weight 10.811. Boron is relatively rare, constituting only 3 ppm of the Earth's crust. It is most commonly found in the borate minerals borax, and kernite. The element was first isolated by Sir Humphry Davy in 1807 and by Joseph Gay-Lussac and Louis Thenard in 1808.

Boron exists in an amorphous form as an extremely hard, blackish brown powder, and in three crystalline forms that look like metals. Crystalline boron is second only to diamond in hardness but is too brittel for use in metals.

ELEMENTS OF THE EARTH
AND THE HUMAN BODY

Research suggests that boron may be nutritionally important. Apparently it helps to maintain appropriate body levels of minerals and horomones needed for bone health.

Uses

The low electrical conductivity of boron increases greatly as its temperature is raised. At certain temperatures, therefore, boron behaves as a semiconductor, and it is often added to germanium and silicon to increase their electrical conductivity. The use of cubic boron nitride as a high-temperature semiconductor is also being explored.

Small additions of boron to steel appreciably increase the hardness of the alloy. Boron is also used in the production of pure, strong metals to remove the oxygen and nitrogen dissolved in the metal or chemically bound to it, and it is used to absorb fast neutrons in nuclear reactors.

The most important boron compound is borax, which has been used in pottery glazes since the Middle Ages. Borax deposits were first found in Tibet, and borax was brought to Europe by the Arabs. It is still important in the ceramic industry. Borax combines with chromium, copper, manganese, cobalt, and nickel to form beautifully colored compounds. Borax beads were once used as a reagent in the detection of these elements.

Borax is also important in the production of borosilicate glass, which has a high refractive index and is suitable for the manufacture of lenses.

Other applications of borax include the impregnation of textiles and wood to make them fire resistant; softening water for laundry; and as a flux in brazing (dissolution of oxides). A weak base, borax is also used in buffer solutions and photographic developers.

Since boron is important in the calcium cycle of plants, borax or boric acid is often added to boron-poor soils as a fertilizer. Boric acid is obtained by the action of strong acids on borax and is used as a mild disinfectant. Although its toxicity is low, it is not completely harmless. Its use as a food preservative is prohibited in many countries.

ELEMENTS OF THE EARTH
AND THE HUMAN BODY

Boron Chemistry

Boron has three valence electrons and forms covalent compounds almost exclusively. It generally forms planar, thre-bonded compounds wiht 120 degree bond angles. These compounds have only six bonding electrons. The boron atom can attain a rare gas configuration, with eight bonding electrons, in reactions of molecules with free electron pairs. Boron forms compounds with nitrogen in a similar way.

BROMINE

The chemical element bromine is a liquid with a powerful, unpleasant odor. Its symbol is Br; its atomic number 35; and its atomic weight 79.904. In its elemental state it is a deep-red color, so dark as to appear almost black. It is a nonmetal appearing on the periodic chart of the elements as a member of family VIIa, the halogens.

Occurrence

In cosmic abundance bromine is 36th among the elements; in the Earth's crust it has been calculated as 48th. At 0.0065 percent by weight, it is the 7th most abundant element dissolved in seawater, gases excepted.

Because of its high reactivity it is never found free in nature, yet neither is it a major constituent in any mineral except a rare silver ore first identified in 1841 near Zacatecas, Mexico. It is more commonly found in underground brines such as those in Michigan and Arkansas and in saline basins such as Searles Lake in California and the Dead Sea. Much is also present in underground salt beds such as those near Stassfurt, East Germany.

Both marine plants and animals are capable of concentrating bromine in their bodies and by doing so become sources of the element. Certain kelp and shellfish are examples, and the fabled Tyrian purple dye was prepared from the bromine-containing secretion of a Mediterranean mollusk, the murex.

ELEMENTS OF THE EARTH
AND THE HUMAN BODY

Chemical Properties

Bromine is similar chemically to chlorine and combines directly with many elements and compounds, but it does so less energetically. It is completely miscible in several organic solvents such as carbon tetrachloride and benzene, which can be used to extract the element from water solutions.

Bromine reacts with most metals, explosively with potassium and vigorously with aluminum, but magnesium, nickel, and lead are unreactive with it. In some cases, as with iron and zinc, moisture must be present to initiate the reaction, and in other cases, as with sodium, an elevated temperature must be attained.

The reaction of bromine with organic compounds is called bromination. Bromine commonly adds across the bond of unsaturated hydrocarbons and reacts with the ring structure of phenol by substitution for hydrogen atoms.

Bromine is an oxidizing agent. It hydrolyzes slightly in aqueous solution, producing hydrobromic acid (HBr) and hypobromous acid (HBrO). The hypobromous acid is unstable, resulting in the production of oxygen, which accounts for the bleaching capability of bromine water. In a freezing mixture of saturated bromine in water, deposits of red crystals of bromine hydrate will form.

Uses

Bromine is chiefly used in the production of dibromoethane, which is added to automotive fuels containing tetraethyl lead. During combustion of the fuel within the automobile engine, the tetraethyl lead forms a volatile lead bromide that becomes part of the exhaust gases, thereby preventing lead buildup within the engine. It is also valuable in dyes, in photographic emulsions, as bleach modifiers, in fire retardants, in disinfectants, in methylene bromide fire extinguishers, and as a mild sedative, hence the term "an old bromide."

Hazards

Bromine is toxic and a severe irritant to the membranes of the respiratory tract and the eyes. It is a powerful oxidizer and may cause ignition of combustible materials upon contact;   thus it is a moderate to high fire hazard.

CALCIUM

The chemical element calcium is a malleable, light, silver-white metal, a member of the alkaline earth metal group. Its symbol is Ca, atomic number 20, and atomic weight 40.08.

Antoine Lavoisier may have been the first chemist to realize that certain metallic oxides exist in nature that cannot be reduced to the pure state by the use of carbon. He suggested that oxides of the alkaline earth metals were among these. Later in the early 19th century, Sir Humphry Davy heated a mixture of lime, CaO, and mercuric oxide, HgO, obtaining very small quantities of an amalgam (mercury alloy) of calcium. Because the quantity was too small to analyze, the element was not discovered until 1808, when Berzelius and Pontin suggested that electrolyzing a mixture of lime and mercury produces an amalgam not then characterized. Davy, using a powerful battery, was able to make this amalgam in sufficient quantity to permit distillation of the mercury, revealing the elemental calcium for the first time.   The name is derived from the mineral CALCITE, a form of calcium carbonate.

Occurrence

In cosmic abundance calcium is 13th among the elements; on Earth it ranks 5th and forms 3.2% of the Earth's crust, being less prevalent than aluminum (7.3%) or iron (4.1%). It is not found free in nature but is common as the carbonate rock limestone. It is also well distributed as the minerals calcium phosphate, silicate, fluoride, and sulfate. As calcium magnesium carbonate it is one of the principal components of dolomite minerals and is found in pearls, coral, natural chalk, calcite, onyx, and marble.

Chemical Properties

Calcium reacts readily as a reducing agent with most nonmetals. It reacts with all halogens and the halide film formed on the surface of large pieces of metal protects the interior atoms from further reaction.

Oxygen behaves similarly. Calcium reacts spontaneously with water and acids to liberate hydrogen gas.

Although heat is required to form calcium nitride, directly from its elements, the reaction occurs very slowly even at ordinary temperatures, resulting in calcium's slow reaction with the nitrogen of the atmosphere. Oxygen has a similar effect, but if they are heated together, calcium burns with a brilliant light.

Biological Functions

Besides being a major mineral in such hard biological structures as shells, bones, and teeth, calcium plays other important roles in the biochemistry of most organisms. In the human body, which consists of about 2 percent calcium by weight, about 99 percent of this calcium occurs in the bones and teeth and the remainder in body cells and fluids. This remainder, however, is essential to muscle contraction and hence to cardiac function. Calcium ions are also essential in the transmission of nerve impulses and in blood coagulation, and their roles in processes such as vision are the subject of ongoing research.

Parathyroid and thyroid hormones help to maintain proper calcium balance in tissues. A lack of calcium can impair growth and lead to such conditions as rickets and tetany. Milk, milk products, leafy green vegetables, and shellfish are sources of dietary calcium.

Calcium absorption

Absorption of calcium occurs mainly in the duodenum by an active process. Vitamin D facilitates calcium absorption as much as four times more than that in vitamin D deficiency states. It is believed that a calcium-binding protein, which increases after vitamin D administration, binds calcium in the intestinal cell during absorption, followed by calcium transfer out of the base of the cell to the blood circulation.

Production

An important method of producing pure calcium is by the reduction of calcium chloride using metallic aluminum. It is also commonly produced by the electrolysis of fused calcium chloride at 800 deg C. As it forms, the light molten calcium metal floats to the surface, where it is continuously withdrawn.

Important Compounds

Because limestone--calcium carbonate--is so abundant in nature and so readily converted to other compounds, it may be regarded as the most important calcium compound. Conversion to other compounds is accomplished by the addition of an acid. Moreover, limestone can be decomposed simply by heating. This is an inexpensive method for the production of lime.

Lime was used even in ancient times; Cato (234-149 BC) wrote of its preparation, properties, and uses. It was used in the mortars during the construction of Rome, and the Greeks also used it. When lime reacts with water in the process called "slaking," 15.96 kcal of heat are liberated for each mole, and calcium hydroxide is formed. Ordinary mortar and some plasters are a mixture of calcium hydroxide, sand, and water. Exposure to air causes evaporation of the water; the mortar hardens, and in the course of time reaction with the carbon dioxide of the atmosphere reforms calcium carbonate, the starting material. Plasters of this material were used in Mesopotamia in 3500 BC.

Calcium fluoride, as fluorspar, is the raw material from which fluorine is derived; calcium chloride, found in salt brines and as a by-product in the Solvay process of production of sodium carbonate, is well known as a dehydrating agent and ice-melting chemical. Calcium sulfate dihydrate is known as gypsum, and a hemihydrate calcium compound is plaster of Paris. Calcium phosphate is converted to superphosphate by the reaction with sulfuric acid and used extensively as a fertilizer.

Calcium carbide is prepared by the reaction of coke and lime in an electric furnace and large quantities are used in the preparation of acetylene, and a fertilizer, cyanamide. Common glass is a mixture of the oxides of sodium, calcium, and silicon in various proportions.

ELEMENTS OF THE EARTH
AND THE HUMAN BODY

CERIUM

Cerium is a chemical element, the most abundant of the lanthanide series. Its symbol is Ce, atomic number 58, and atomic weight 140.12. It occurs in many minerals, especially monazite and bastnaesite. The element was discovered in 1803 by M. H. Klaproth and independently by J. J. Berzelius and W. Hisinger. It was named after Ceres, an asteroid. Finely divided cerium, which may ignite spontaneously, is a constituent of an iron alloy used for lighter flints. Cerium and misch metal, an alloy of 50 percent cerium with several other rare earth metals, are used to remove oxygen in vacuum tubes.

CESIUM

Cesium is a chemical element, a soft, silver-white alakal metal. Its symbol is Cs, its atomic number 55, and its atomic weight 132.905. The element was discovered by Robert Bunsen and Gustav Kirchhoff in 1860. The stable isotope Cs-133 occurs naturally. Many radioactive isotopes have been produced artificially; Cs-137, with a half-life of 33 years, is used as a source of gamma radiation. Cesium reacts violently with water, and may ignite spontaneously on exposure to moist air. Because of its sensitivity to light, it is used in photoelectric devices. It is used to remove traces of gas in vacuum tubes. The natural frequency of the cesium atom is used as a time standard in the cesium clock, a type of atomic clock.

CHROMIUM

The chemical element chromium is a lustrous metal of the transition series. Its chemical symbol is Cr, atomic numer 24, and atomic weight 51.996. Chromium was discovered in 1798 by N. L. Vauquelin. Its name is derived from the Greek word for color, since most chromium compounds are brightly colored. Chromium does not occur free innature; in bound form it makes up 0.1-0.3 parts per million of the Earth'scrust. The only important chromium ore is chromite. The red color of rubies and

171

the green color of emeralds, serpentine, and chrome mica are caused by chromium.

Preparation.

Chromium metal is prepared by reducing the ore in a blast furnace with carbon (coke) or silicon to form an alloy of chromium and iron called ferrochrome, which is used as the starting material for the many iron-containing alloys that use chromium. Chromium to be used in iron-free alloys is obtained by reduction or electrolysis of chromium compounds. Chromium is difficult to work in the pure metal form; it is brittle at low temperatures, and its high melting point (1,900 deg C/3, 452 deg F) makes it difficult to cast.

Uses.

The most important use of chromium is in chrome plating, which creates a hard, wear-resistant, attractive surface. Chrome plating can be performed by immersion or by electrolysis. The latter method allows very thin layers to be deposited but uses a good deal of current; the cathode current efficiency is only 10-15 percent.

Chromium is alloyed with iron to improve its resistance to corrosion, its hardness, and its workability. Other metals, such as vanadium, manganese, tungsten, and molybdenum, are added to these alloys in order to obtain special properties. Genuine stainless steel always contains nickel and chromium. Super corrosion-resistant types of steel, such as those used for furnaces, heat exchangers, and burner heads, contain about 30 percent chromium.

Important nonferrous (iron-free) chromium alloys include stellite, which contains cobalt and tungsten and is used in cutting, lathing, and milling tools; and nickel-chromium (nichrome), which is used in resistance wire in electrical heaters, irons, and toasters.

Compounds.

The most important valences of chromium are 3 and 6, although chromium with valences of 1, 2, 4, and 5 has also been shown to exist in a number of compounds. Chromium compounds often have a green color, but yellow, blue, red, and violet compounds are also known. The most important one is chromic oxide, which is used as a pigment (chromic oxide green). Chrome alum forms beautiful violet crystals and is used in the tanning of leather and in textile dyeing. A number of other chromium salts are also used in the textile industry as mordants. Chromium compounds with a valence of 6 are called chromates; most have a yellow color and all are toxic. When absorbed into the body they severely irritate the gastrointestinal tract, leading to circulatory shock and renal damage. Chromate yellow, one of the most important yellow pigments, is highly toxic because it contains both chromium and lead. Chromates are used as anticorrodents in water-cooling systems. Unfortunately, because they are toxic, their runoff has severe effects on river flora. It is economically and ecologically wise to remove chromates before waste water is released.

In 1959, traces of chromium were shown to be required for health as part of a still somewhat elusive "glucose tolerance factor". Apart from its role in glucose metabolism, chromium is presumably also involved in lipid and cholesterol metabolism.

COBALT

The chemical element cobalt is a hard silver metal with a bluish sheen. Its chemical symbol is Co, its atomic number is 27, and its atomic weight is 58.9332. Cobalt is a transition element with chemical properties like those of iron and nickel.

Occurrence.

Cobalt is 0.001% to 0.002% of the Earth's crust. Never found in pure form, cobalt is usually bonded to arsenic and sulfur. The best-known cobalt minerals are cobaltite (cobalt glance); linnaeite (cobalt pyrite); smaltite; and erythrite. Cobalt is also a constituent of many meteorites and is found in the Sun and the atmospheres of stars.

The name cobalt, derived from the German kobold (a malicious underground goblin or demon), originated in the 16th century, when arsenic-containing cobalt ores were dug up in silver mines of the Harz Mountains. Believing that the ores contained copper, miners heated them and were injured by the toxic arsenic trioxide vapors that were released.

ELEMENTS OF THE EARTH
AND THE HUMAN BODY

Uses.

Cobalt is a relatively expensive metal used in the manufacture of valuable alloys. Cobalt-iron alloys have special magnetic properties; for example, Hyperco is used as the nucleus for strong electromagnets. Alloys of titanium, aluminum, cobalt, and nickel, such as alnico and ticonal, can be made permanently magnetic. Stellite, an alloy of cobalt, chromium, tungsten, and molybdenum, is very hard and retains its hardness even at high temperatures. It is used in cutting tools, combustion-engine valves, and parts for gas turbines. Stone saws are sometimes manufactured from cobalt in which very hard particles of tungsten and titanium carbides have been occluded.

Cobalt Isotopes. Co-59 is the only naturally-occurring cobalt isotope. Other isotopes, all of them radioactive, have been artificially produced. Among these, Co-60, which is normally produced by irradiating Co-59 with neutrons in an atomic reactor, is especially important.

Natural cobalt is often added to hydrogen bombs; upon explosion, many neutrons are liberated, which convert the cobalt to Co-60, causing a considerable increase in the total amount of radioactive fallout. Co-60 is also used in cancer research and as a source of X rays for radiation therapy.

Chemical Properties.

Chemically, cobalt resembles iron and nickel. Iron is situated to its left and nickel to its right in the periodic table. These three metals constitute the iron group. The most common valence of cobalt is +2; trivalent cobalt salts are usually strong oxidizing agents, and a valence of +4 occurs in rare instances. Cobalt salts have a strong tendency to form coordination compounds. Because cobalt forms such compounds with carbon monoxide, CO, cobalt salts are often used as catalysts in chemical processes involving carbon monoxide. Most trivalent cobalt complexes dissolve poorly in water, making it easier to separate cobalt from nickel. Many coordination compounds of cobalt are intensely colored; several of them are used as dyes, such as Thenard's blue; Fischer's salt, or cobalt yellow; cobalt blue; and cobalt red. The color of some cobalt salts depends on the number of molecules of water of crystallization present. Thus, cobalt(II) chloride varies from dark violet to light red. This salt can be used as an "invisible" ink. A pink solution of cobalt chloride is practically colorless when dry; when heated, the water of crystallization evaporates and the ink turns violet blue. Formerly, these salts were classified according to their color: luteo salts, yellow; roseo salts, red; and purpureo salts, violet.

Cobalt seems to be essential to life. It is especially important in animal nutrition. A deficiency of vitamin B-12, which is a cobalt compound, can cause pernicious anemia.

Prior to World War II, Australian workers associated a lock of cobalt in the pastures with a condition in cattle known as "wasting" or "coast disease" (Underwood and Filmer, 1935). While mildly affected animals show no symptoms other than a nonspecific unthriftiness, it is fatal in the acute form, leading to rapid wasting, anemia, and death. The disease can be prevented by the addition of traces of inorganic cobalt slats to the feedstock or pastures but was eventually recognized to be caused by vitamin B_{12} rather than cobalt efficiency (Smith et al., 1951). The discovery of the presence of one atom of tightly bound cobalt in the molecule of vitamin B_{12} added new dimensions to trace element research, especially after vitamin B_{12} coenzyme was shown to be a compound with a direct cobalt-carbon bond (Lenhert and Crowfoot-Hodgkin, 1961). The corrinoid coenzyme is one of the most efficient biocatalysts known, effecting unusual molecular rearrangements in a number of enzymes.

COPPER

The chemical element copper is a reddish metal at the head of group IB in the periodic table. Its symbol is Cu; atomic number, 29; and atomic weight, 63.546. Copper follows the first transitional series of elements, and its positive ion, displays transitional properties.

Copper was the first metal used by humans and is second only to iron in its utility through the ages. The name is derived from the Latin cuprum, "copper," from the earlier Latin Cyprium, "Cyprian metal." The discovery of the metal dates from prehistoric times, and it is estimated that copper was first used about 5000 BC or even earlier.

ELEMENTS OF THE EARTH
AND THE HUMAN BODY

Physical and Chemical Properties

Eleven isotopes of copper are known, two of which are not radioactive and occur with a natural abundance of 69.09% and 30.91%, respectively. Copper melts at 1,083.4 deg plus or minus 0.2 deg C (in a vacuum), boils at 2,567 deg C, and has a density of 8.96 at 20 deg C. The element has a hardness of 3, takes on a bright metallic luster, has a cubic crystal structure, and is malleable, ductile, and a good conductor of heat and electricity, second only to silver in electrical conductivity.

Copper exhibits oxidation states of +2 (the most common, forming Cu(II) compounds), and +1 (Cu(I), stable only in aqueous solution if part of a stable complex ion); a few compounds of copper(III) are also known. Although the electronic configuration of copper is formally similar to that of the alkali metals (Group IA) in general and potassium in particular, the behavior of copper is considerably different from that of the alkali metals. The shielding of the outer electron from the attraction of the nucleus is stronger than in copper. Thus the outer electron in copper is more tightly bound, resulting in a comparatively high first ionization potential and a relatively small ionic radius for copper.

The outstanding feature of copper and the other metals of Group IB (gold and silver) is their resistance to chemical attack. Copper is slowly attacked by moist air, and its surface gradually becomes covered with the characteristic green patina that consists of basic sulfate. At about 300 deg C copper is attacked by air or oxygen, and a black coating of copper(II) oxide forms at the surface; at a temperature of 1,000 deg C copper(I) oxide is formed instead. The metal is attacked by sulfur vapor, with the formation of copper(I) sulfide; and by the halogens, which form copper(II) halides, except iodine, which forms copper(I) iodide. Copper is not attacked by water or steam, and dilute nonoxidizing acids, such as dilute hydrochloric and dilute sulfuric acids, have no effect in the absence of an oxidizing agent. The metal is attacked by boiling concentrated hydrochloric acid with the evolution of hydrogen, by hot concentrated sulfuric acid, and by dilute or concentrated nitric acid.

Alloys of Copper

Copper mixes well with many elements, and more than 1,000 different alloys have been formed, several of which are technologically significant. The presence of the other element or elements can modify the hot or cold machining properties, tensile strength, corrosion fatigue, and wear resistance of the copper; it is also possible to create alloys of pleasing colors.

Relationship to Life Sciences

Copper is a trace element essential to the healthy life of many plants and animals, in which it usually occurs as part of the oxidizing enzymes such as ascorbic acid oxidase, tyrosinase, lactase, and monoamine oxidase. These enzymes, which are high-molecular-weight proteins containing 0.05%-0.35% of Cu, play an important part in living oxidation and reduction reactions, in which the copper undergoes cyclic changes between Cu(I) and Cu(II) oxidation states. The metal is tightly bound to ligand sites, containing oxygen, sulfur, or nitrogen atoms on the protein.

The hereditary deficiency of the protein ceruloplasmin, known as Wilson's disease, is associated with a pathological increase in the copper content of almost all tissues, particularly the brain and liver. Albino mammals lack the normal form of the copper-containing enzyme tyrosinase, which participates in the synthesis of the pigment melanin. Copper can be toxic in large quantities, especially to lower organisms such as bacilli, fungi, and algae.

Applications of Copper and Its Compounds

The electrical industry is a major consumer of copper. The metal is used for the windings of generators and for conveying electrical power. Its resistance to chemical attack and its high thermal conductivity make copper a useful metal for condensers in chemical plants and for car radiators. Copper tubing is widely employed in plumbing, and finely divided copper is used as an industrial catalyst in the oxidation of methanol to formaldehyde. Copper compounds, such as Fehling solution, are used in analytical tests for sugars.

As late as the early 1920s copper was suggested because of the basis of empirical evidence, to be of value in the diet of rats.(Bodansky, 1921). It was later discovered that copper is required for the formation of aortic elastin (O'Dell et al., 1961), and thus is of crucial importance for heart functioning. Copper deficient laboratory animals have since been found to exhibit glucose intolerance and abnormalities in cardiac function. Deficient animals may die suddenly with a ruptured heart, caused by thinning of the aortic wall. These findings have ominous significance in light of recent copper estimates in typical human diets in the United States; 75% of the diets examined furnished less that 2 mg of copper per day, the amount thought to be required by adults (Klevay, 1982).

DYSPROSIUM

The element dysprosium is a silver gray rare-earth metal in group IIIB of the periodic table. Its symbol is Dy, atomic number 66, and atomic weight 162.50. The element was identified in 1886 but was not isolated until 1950. Its name is derived from the Greek word dysprositos, meaning "difficulty of access." Seven isotopes occur naturally. Dysprosium has a valence of + 3. Its oxide, Dy2 03, is used in control devices for nuclear reactors because the metal has a high neutron-absorbing capability, and in cryogenic cooling devices because it is one of the most paramagnetic substances known.

ERBIUM

Erbium is a chemical element, a shiny metal of the lanthanide series. Its symbol is Er, its atomic number 68, and its atomic weight 167.26. The six naturally occurring erbium isotopes--Er-162, Er-164, Er-166, Er-167, Er-168, and Er-170--are not radioactive. The numerous synthetic isotopes of erbium are all radioactive. Erbium was first identified in nature by C. G. Mosander in 1842. Because of its capacity to absorb neutrons, erbium is widely used in manufacturing nuclear control rods. It is also used in magnetic alloys.

EUROPIUM

Europium is a chemical element, a metal of the lanthanide series. Its symbol is Eu; its atomic number is 63; and its atomic weight is 151.96. Two isotopes of europium occur naturally, Eu-151 and Eu-153; both are stable. Many radioactive, artificial isotopes of europium have been created. The existence of europium was first postulated by Sir William Crookes in

1889. In 1896, E. A. Demarcay discovered element 63 and named it for Europe. Europium, a soft metal, is the most reactive of the lanthanides, and many of its properties are more like those of calcium, strontium, and barium. Europium oxide is used as the red phosphor in cathode-ray tubes for color television receivers. Because europium easily absorbs neutrons, it is used in control rods for nuclear reactors.

FLUORINE

Fluorine is a pale yellow, poisonous, highly corrosive gas. It is the lightest member of the halogens and the most reactive of all elements. Its symbol is F, its atomic weight is 18.99840, and its atomic number is 9. The name fluorine is derived from the mineral fluorspar, which, in turn, is derived from the Latin fluo ("flow"), because until AD 1500 it was used as a flux in metallurgy.

Natural Occurence

Fluorine is widely distributed among natural compounds, but its extreme reactivity precludes its presence in elemental form. Although constituting only 0.065 percent of the Earth's crust, fluorine is found in oceans, lakes, rivers, and all other forms of natural water; in the bones, teeth, and blood of all mammals; and in all plants and plant parts. In spite of its ubiquity, as yet no universally acceptable evidence exists that fluorine is a necessary ingredient of living beings. Fluorine is found most abundantly in nature as the minerals fluorspar (fluorite, cryolite, and fluorapatite. Fluorspar is found extensively in Illinois and Kentucky. Cryolite occurs extensively in Greenland and Iceland, although its use in the production of aluminum is so extensive that much of the supply needed for other manufacturing must be produced synthetically. Of the three minerals, fluorapatite is the most abundant.

Properties

Fluorine exists as a diatomic gas. Highly toxic, it has a characteristic pungent odor that can be detected before hazardous concentrations build up. Fluorine boils at-188 deg C (- 370 deg F) and its melting point is - 219 deg C (- 426 deg F).

Only one stable isotope of fluorine occurs. The fluorine atom has seven electrons in its outer shell and requires an additional electron for maximum stability. This electron is strongly attracted by the positively charged nucleus because of the small size of the fluorine atom, accounting for the extreme electronegativity of the element. As a result, fluorine has a valance of -1 and forms compounds with all elements except the noble gases helium, neon, and argon. Fluorine salts are called fluorides.

Fluorine is manufactured by electrolyzing a mixture of potassium fluoride and hydrogen fluoride. It is stored and shipped in containers lined with Teflon or made of a special steel. The latter becomes coated with iron fluoride, thus retarding further reaction.

Uses and compounds

In addition to its use in uranium processing, refrigerants, and aerosol propellants, fluorine is used in dentifrices, as a catalyst in producing the dodecylbenzene used to make detergents, and in alkylating olefins used in refining high-octane gasoline, as well as in the production of polyfluorhydrocarbon resins such as Teflon, noted for their nonstick properties and resistance to corrosion.

Sodium fluoride, NaF, is used as a sterilant, an insecticide, and a water-treatment agent in fluoridating municipal supplies. It is also a paint preservative, it renders enamels opaque, and it is used in dyes and in the primary metal and ceramics industries. Boron trifluoride is a catalyst in the alkylation of benzene for detergent production and in making polymers and copolymers for adhesives.

Other chemically important compounds of fluorine are antimony trifluoride, an organic chemistry catalyst; sulfur hexafluoride, a gaseous insulator; and several polymers such as vinylidene fluoride. Fluorine compounds are of interest whenever incombustibility or oil and water resistance are important. They are also used in elastomers and in surfactants for the preparation of coatings applied to fiberboard, paper, and cloth.

The addition of 1.5-2.0 ppm of Fluoride   produced a definite enhancement of longitutinal growth in young rats during the first 4 weeks of post natal life.   In other experiments, fluoride-deficient female mice developed diminished fertility and became anemic.   As to the toxicity of fluoride, it is remarkable that diets containing even 300-500 ppm fluoride may be administered to laboratory animals for prolonged periods of time without causing apparent harm.   Fluoride in the water, on the other hand, produces a characteristic mottling of the enamel of permanent teeth at concentrations as low as 1.5 ppm.   At 1ppm, the concentration at which fluoride is added to some drinking water supplies, mottling does not occur, while the anticariogenic effects are optimal.

GADOLINIUM

The chemical element gadolinium is a lustrous, magnetic metal of the rare earth lanthanide series, group IIIB of the periodic table.   Its symbol is Gd, its atomic number 64, its atomic weight 157.25, and its valence +3. It is often found in association with other rare earths. Gadolinium oxide was isolated in 1880 by the French chemist J. C. G. de Marignac from the mineral gadolinite, for which the element is named. Seven gadolinium isotopes occur in nature.   At least one, 152Gd, is radioactive, with a half-life of 1.1×10 to the 14th power in years.   With the highest neutron-absorption cross-section of any known element, gadolinium is used in control rods in some nuclear reactors.   It is also used in noise filters, in phosphors for color television, and to increase the tensile strength and electrical conductivity of some other metals.

GALLIUM

The chemical element gallium is a bluish metal of group IIIA in the periodic table.   Its chemical symbol is Ga, atomic number 31, and atomic weight 69.72.

Gallium is a relatively rare metal that is becoming increasingly important in the manufacture of semiconductor electronic devices.   Its existence was originally detected spectroscopically; it was isolated for the first time from zinc sulfide ore in 1875 by the French chemist Lecoq de

ELEMENTS OF THE EARTH
AND THE HUMAN BODY

Boisbaudran, who named it after Gallia, the Latin name for France. Later the same year, Dmitry Mendeleyev showed that gallium was the missing group IIIA element below aluminum and above indium predicted in his theory of chemical periodicity.

Gallium is present in the earth's crust in an average abundance of 5-15 ppm. It often occurs in small amounts in the sulfide ores of its neighbors in the periodic table, zinc and germanium, and, because of its chemical similarity to aluminum, it is a minor component in all aluminum ores. It is not present in significant concentration in the ocean. No important mineral deposits contain a high percentage of gallium.

Most of the world's gallium is produced in the United States. The metal is recovered by controlled electrolysis of the concentrated alkaline liquors that are by-products of the extraction of aluminum and zinc from their ores. Ultrapure gallium (99.9999%) for semiconductor electronics is obtained by repeated fractional crystallization of the metal. Gallium is relatively expensive because of its low concentration in most minerals and because the metal must be extremely pure for most applications.

The pure metal has a slight bluish luster resembling that of zinc. Its melting point (29.78 deg C) is unusually low, and the boiling point (about 2,250 deg C) is not precisely known because the metal is highly active at high temperature. For this reason most of the expected applications of the low melting point and exceptional 2,200 deg liquid range, such as use in thermometers and related devices, are impractical. Molten gallium expands in volume by 3.2% on freezing; among all the other elements only bismuth shares this property.

Gallium normally forms compounds in the trivalent state. A +1 state also exists, but it is easily oxidized to gallium(III). A rare +2 state has been reported, but all gallium(II) compounds are unstable. At room temperature the metal is kept from corroding in air by a protective oxide film. Corrosion occurs rapidly at high temperature, however, because the metal reduces the oxide film to a state which evaporates to constantly expose a fresh surface. Hot molten gallium forms alloys with most other metals, severely restricting such practical applications as serving as a high temperature substitute for mercury.

The most important gallium compounds are the semiconductors, formed with the elements phosphorus, arsenic, and antimony. The most widely used and studied compound is gallium arsenide, GaAs, which has a number of electronic properties possessed by neither germanium nor silicon and has important applications in solid-state microwave generators and photoelectric cells. It is also used in lasers, because the light emitted from GaAs diodes (electroluminescence) is coherent and has a narrow frequency bandwidth. Gallium compounds have no known biological function, and ordinary gallium salts have very low toxicity.

GERMANIUM

The chemical element germanium, semimetal of group IVA in the periodic table, is of central importance in the manufacture of semiconductor materials and devices. Its symbol is Ge, atomic number 32, and atomic weight 72.59. The German chemist Clemens A. Winkler first isolated the element in 1886 from the mineral argyrodite, a mixed sulfide of silver and germanium, and named it after his homeland. Germanium is widely distributed in the Earth's crust, with an average abundance of about 7 grams per metric ton. The element is usually found as a minor component in sulfide ores of copper, zinc, tin, lead, and antimony.

Germanium has a brittle metallic appearance, a melting point of 937.4 deg C, and a boiling point of 2,830 deg C. It crystallizes in a cubic structure similar to diamond but has a hardness of only 6 on Moh's scale (diamond is 10). The ultrapure element is an intrinsic semiconductor, which accounts for its major use in solid-state electronics. It forms compounds in the +2 and +4 oxidation states. The +2 state is both easily reduced to the element and easily oxidized to Ge(IV), so that tetravalent germanium compounds are the most common. The chloride and oxide germanium tetrachloride and germaium dioxide are the most important compounds because of the role they play in the production of the pure element.

Ultrapure germanium can be produced in near-crystalline perfection more easily than other semiconductors. For this reason alone, the electronic properties of germanium have been studied more than those of any other solid. The earliest semiconductor research was done with this element, and William Shockley used germanium to make the first transistor in 1948.

ELEMENTS OF THE EARTH
AND THE HUMAN BODY

Germanium is recovered by treating enriched wastes and residues from zinc sulfide ores, pyrometallic ores, and coal with hydrochloric acid to form the volatile liquid which is extracted with carbon tetrachloride and purified by distillation. The tetrachloride is treated with demineralized water to precipitate the dioxide which is then reduced to germanium with hydrogen. The ultrapure element is obtained by zone refining, a selective fusion-recrystallization process that concentrates impurities in the melt.

Germanium dioxide is finding increasing use in special optical materials. Fused dioxide glasses have transmission characteristics greatly superior to quartz glasses in the infrared portion of the spectrum.

GOLD

The chemical element gold, atomic number 79, symbol Au (from the Latin aurum), is a soft, lustrous yellow, malleable metal. It is one of the transition metals and its atomic weight is 196.967.

Occurence

Although the Earth's crust averages a mere 0.004 grams of gold per ton, commercial concentrations of gold are found in areas distributed widely over the globe. Gold occurs in association with ores of copper and lead, in quartz veins, in the gravel of stream beds, and with pyrites (iron sulfide). Seawater contains astonishing quantities of gold, but so much energy is required for its recovery that the process is not economical. The ancients found quantities of gold in Ophir, Sheba, Uphaz, Parvaim, Arabia, India, and Spain. By the time of Christ, written reports were made of deposits in Thracia, Italy, and Anatolia. Gold is also found in Wales, in Hungary, in the Ural Mountains of Russia, and, in large quantities, in Australia.

The distribution of gold seems to validate the theory that gold was carried toward the Earth's surface from great depths by geologic activity, perhaps with other metals as a solid solution within molten rock. After this solid solution cooled, its gold content was spread through such a great volume of rock that large fragments were unusual; this theory explains why much of the world's gold is in small, often microscopic particles. The theory also explains why small amounts of gold are widespread in all

ELEMENTS OF THE EARTH
AND THE HUMAN BODY

igneous rocks; they are rarely chemically combined and seldom in quantities rich enough to be called an ore.

Because of its poor chemical reactivity, gold was one of the first two or three metals (along with copper and silver) used by humans in its elemental state. Because it is relatively unreactive, it was found uncombined and required no previously developed knowledge of refining. Its first uses are unknown, but it was probably used in decorative arts before 9000 BC. Even civilizations that developed little or no use of other metals prized gold for its beauty.

Gold is the most malleable of all metals. It can be beaten into sheets approaching a single atom of thickness, so thin as to transmit light.

Chemical properties

Gold forms amalgams with several metals, is readily alloyed, and can be dissolved in aqua regia and a few other solvents. It is, however, poorly reactive, which explains why it is generally found as a free metal. Nevertheless, both aurous (gold I) and auric (gold III) compounds are known, as are coordination compounds in which gold is apparently the central metal atom.

Extration and refining

In obtaining gold from vein ore, the ore is first crushed in rod or ball mills. This process reduces the ore to a powdery substance from which the gold can be extracted by amalgamation with mercury or by placer procedures. About 70% is recovered at this point. The remainder is dissolved in dilute solutions of sodium cyanide or calcium cyanide. The addition of metallic zinc to these solutions causes metallic gold to precipitate. This precipitate is refined by smelting. The purification is completed by electrolysis similar to that previously described for copper, and the sludge produced will contain commercial quantities of silver, platinum, osmium, and other rare-earth metals.

Uses

The largest single use of gold today is as currency or currency reserves. Gold is the one substance universally accepted in exchange for goods or services. There is also a large and rapidly growing demand for gold in industrial processes. Its relatively high electrical conductivity and extremely high resistance to corrosion make the metal critically important in microelectrical circuits. Minute quantities dissolved in glass or plastic sheets prevent the passage of infrared radiation and make an efficient heat shield. Because of its chemical stability, gold is in demand for bearings used in corrosive atmospheres. It is also plated on surfaces exposed to corrosive fluids or vapors. Many other industrial uses demand the properties unique to gold. Its lack of toxicity and its compatability with living systems make it indispensable in dentistry and medicine, and its beauty has made it outstanding in the arts and crafts since the beginning of written history.

HOLMIUM

Holmium is a silvery, soft metal of the rare earths, or lanthanide series of chemical elements. Its symbol is Ho, its atomic number 67, its atomic weight 164.93, and its group IIIB. The only naturally occurring isotope, Ho-165, is stable. Holmium forms salts with oxygen, chlorine, bromine, and iodine. It was discovered in 1878 by J. L. Soret and M. Delafontaine and independently by Per Teodor Cleve (1879), who named it for the city of Stockholm.

IODINE

Iodine, atomic number 53, symbol I, is a solid nonmetallic element of the halogen family, a group that includes the elements fluorine, chlorine, and bromine. At room temperature iodine is a lustrous, blue-black, crystalline solid of atomic weight 126.9045.

Iodine is the least water-soluble halogen, but its solubility is appreciably increased in aqueous solutions of sodium iodide, due to the formation of polyiodide complex ions. It dissolves readily in alcohol, chloroform, carbon tetrachloride, and benzene.

Occurrence

ELEMENTS OF THE EARTH
AND THE HUMAN BODY

Iodine is the 44th most abundant element in the cosmos, the 62d most abundant in the Earth's crust, and the 17th most abundant of those dissolved in seawater (gases excluded). Although scarce, iodine is widely distributed in nature, occurring in underground brines, rocks, soils, and essentially all living material even though apparently not necessary for life. Because of this general distribution and its low abundance, no large deposits of iodine exist; however, several living systems are able to concentrate it within themselves, thus becoming important sources. Examples are the sea plants and algae such as the Laminaria family. Because of the magnitude of the deposits, the Chilean nitrates, in which it is an impurity, are also important sources of iodine.

Chemical Properties

Like all members of the halogen family iodine is very reactive, although it is somewhat less reactive than the other halogens. Both bromine and chlorine react to liberate free iodine from aqueous solutions of iodides. Iodine vapor reacts directly with most metals to form metal iodides, similar to its reaction with nickel. Iodine also reacts with water, although the reverse reaction predominates at equilibrium.

Iodine reacts with hydrogen sulfide (H(2)S) to liberate sulfur. Its reaction with phosphorus, arsenic, and antimony is similar to that with bismuth. Oxygen compounds of iodine have been prepared also. The several oxidation states available in iodine, -1, +1, +3, +5, and +7, help explain the interhalogen compounds (halogens combined with halogens) all of which are stable at room temperature.

Production

Iodine may be prepared in the laboratory by distilling potassium iodide (KI) or sodium iodide (NaI) with sulfuric acid and manganese dioxide or by the reaction of potassium iodate or sodium iodate with potassium iodide and sulfuric acid. Commercial iodine is produced principally (50%) from Chilean nitrate deposits containing about 0.2% calcium iodate as an impurity. Iodine is recovered from solutions of the nitrate using sodium bisulfite as a reducing agent. Other significant sources of iodine are underground brines such as those found in Michigan. The seaweeds that are able to concentrate the element are now less important in the United States but are still major sources of iodine in some countries.

Uses

The principal use of iodine is in the health sciences. Almost from the year of its discovery it has been used to prevent goiter and now does so by the widespread use of sodium or potassium iodide additives to common table salt. Tincture of iodine has been used as a disinfectant, although iodine complexes now predominate in this application. Iodine complexed with surfactants are used in common sanitizers. Radioactive iodine has found important use in tracer studies, including studies of the thyroid gland.

Other uses of iodine include its use in photographic papers, as tracers used to study stereochemistry, in dyes, as a catalyst, as an indicator in analytic chemistry, in engraving, in special soaps and lubricants, to seed clouds in rainmaking experiments, and as a measure of the degree of unsaturation of organic compounds.

IRON

Iron, a silvery white solid metal, appears in Group VIII of the periodic table as a transion element. Its atomic number is 26, and its atomic weight is 55.847. Its chemical symbol, Fe, is derived from ferrum, the Latin word for iron. Iron is notable among the elements in the abundance of its ores and the vast number of useful alloys that can be formulated with iron as the major constituent. Iron is also biologically important; it is the central atom in heme, the oxygen-carrying portion of hemoglobin found in blood. Elemental iron has been known since prehistoric times. Although how early humans first learned to extract the element from its ores is still debated, scientists are fairly certain that early, highly prized samples of iron were obtained from meteors. Several references to "the metal of heaven"--probably iron--have been found in ancient writings. By approximately 1200 BC, iron was being obtained from its ores; this achievement marks the beginning of the iron age. Even with the dependence today on plastics, concrete, aluminum, and fiberglass, iron and its alloys remain crucial in the economies of modern countries.

ELEMENTS OF THE EARTH
AND THE HUMAN BODY

Occurence

In its various compounds, iron is the fourth most abundant element (5.1%) in the Earth's crust. Evidence exists that the molten core of the Earth is primarily elemental iron. Iron has four natural isotopes; the most abundant has a mass of 56 (91.66%); the latter occurs with isotopes having masses of 54 (5.82%), 57 (2.19%), and 58 (0.33%). Iron occasionally occurs naturally in its pure or uncombined form, but is abundant in combination with other elements, as oxides, sulfides, carbonates, and silicates. Iron ores are naturally occurring compounds of iron from which the metal can easily be recovered in significant quantity. Iron pyrite is a yellow, crystalline mineral called fool's gold because of its goldlike appearance.

Physical Properties

In its pure form, iron is rather soft and is malleable and ductile at room temperature. It melts at 1,535 deg C and boils at 3,000 deg C. Pure iron can exist in two structural types, or allotropic forms. At room temperature, the iron atoms are arranged in a body-centered cubic lattice called the a-form, which is transformed at 910 deg C into a cubic close-packed structure called the gamma-form, (designated by the Greek lower-case letter gamma). At 1,390 deg C iron returns to a body-centered cubic structure, called the delta-form designated by the Greek lower-case letter delta). Iron at room temperature exhibits ferromagnetism, a strong magnetic behavior that the metal may retain even in the absence of an external, applied magnetic field. When iron is heated to 768 deg C, it loses this property and exhibits paramagnetism, a weaker attraction to an applied magnetic field. Between 768 deg and 910 deg C, iron is said to be in its beta-form (designated by the Greek letter beta), which is not a different allotropic form of iron. Although pure iron does conduct electricity, compared to other metals used for that purpose, such as copper or aluminum, it is a poor conductor.

Chemical Properties

Easily oxidized, iron reacts directly with most common nonmetallic elements, forming compounds in which iron is in the +2 or +3 oxidation state. At high temperatures, iron also absorbs hydrogen and nitrogen and forms phosphides, carbides, and silicides. In the absence of water, and under various conditions, iron reacts with oxygen. Finely divided iron burns in air once it is ignited. Larger pieces of iron react with oxygen in dry air at temperatures above 150 deg C to form mixed oxides. At temperatures above 575 deg C and at low concentrations of oxygen, FeO is formed.

Corrosion.

Perhaps the most important chemical reaction of iron, at least from an economic standpoint, is the least desirable one: the reaction of iron, water, and oxygen to form hydrated iron oxide, or rust. The corrosion of iron has been studied carefully, and the formation of rust is known to be an electrochemical reaction. For rust to form at room temperature, three components in addition to iron must be present: oxygen, water, and an electrolyte (an ionic substance dissolved in the water). Iron that is partially immersed in salt or fresh water usually rusts more rapidly than does iron that is totally immersed. In the atmosphere, the formation of rust begins when the relative humidity exceeds 50%. The presence of air pollutants, particularly the oxides of sulfur, greatly increases the rate at which rust forms. In the presence of air and water, sulfur dioxide forms sulfuric acid that attacks and oxidizes the iron. Because rust on the surface of iron is porous, the metal surface beneath the rust also reacts. The formation of rust may be inhibited by coating the surface of the metal with paint or certain other chemicals, or by covering the metal with another metal such as zinc (galvanized iron) or tin (the derivation of "tin" cans).

Aqueous Solutions.

The chemistry of iron in the +2 or the +3 oxidation state is complex; many oxidizing and reducing agents are capable of interconverting its various compounds. For example, the reactions of a solution of potassium ferrocyanide with iron in the +3 oxidatin state and a solution of potassium ferricyanide with iron in the +2 oxidation state both yield a dark blue solid. The product of the first reaction is called Prussian blue, and the other, Turnbull's blue; both have identical compositions. Solutions of iron ions exhibit various chemical and physical properties characteristic of many transition metals. When ferrous sulfate (iron in the +2 oxidation state is called ferrous iron) is dissolved in water, the pale green ferrous hydrate ion is formed. When ferric nitrate (iron in the +3 oxidation state is called ferric iron) is dissolved, the product is the pale violet ferric hydrate ion, which differs from the former ion only by having one less electron. Like most iron ions in solution, both ions are paramagnetic; that is, solutions containing them are attracted by external fields. A seemingly endless number of chemical compounds, both ions and neutral molecules, can replace the water molecules associated with iron in solution. If cyanide ions are added to solutions of the ions mentioned above, the products are ferrocyanide ion and ferricyanide ion, respectively. A change in the magnetic properties of iron occurs when ferrocyanide is formed. Solutions containing this ion are diamagnetic; that is, they are weakly repelled by a magnetic field. By contrast, solutions of the ferric compound are weakly paramagnetic. Iron in the +6 oxidation state can be made by reacting solutions of ferric ion with strong oxidizing agents to produce a reddish purple ion of 1 iron and 4 oxygen atoms, having a double-negative charge and which is also weakly paramagnetic. Organometallic Compounds. Iron in its various oxidation states readily combines with many carbon compounds to form organometallic compounds. Finely divided iron reacts with carbon monoxide under pressure to form the yellow liquid iron pentacarbonyl. This transition metal carbonyl, like many others, contains the metal in a zero oxidation state. The compound is the starting material for thousands of iron compounds in unusually low oxidation states (including some that are formally negative). On decomposition, iron pentacarbonyl yields samples of very pure iron. A new type of organometallic compound was discovered in 1951. If ferrous chloride is reacted with cyclopentadiene in the presence of a strong organic base, the orange crystalline compound ferrocene is the product. This compound, which has a highly stable structure, is called a "sandwich" compound because the iron atom is strongly held between the two flat $C(5)H(5)$ rings. In this case, it is not useful to attempt to assign an oxidation state to iron. The characterization of this compound has led to extensive transition metal organometallic chemistry.

Alloys

Iron is abundant and easily obtainable from its ores. Its desirable mechanical and magnetic properties, as well as its resistance to corrosion, may be improved by mixing iron with other elements, frequently metals, to form alloys, substances that may be simple mixtures of elements; solid solutions, in which the atoms of one substance occupy definite positions relative to the other substances; or as intermetallic compounds. Perhaps the most important alloy of iron is steel, which contains up to approximately 2% carbon. Steels that contain about 0.25% carbon are called mild steels; those with about 0.45% carbon are medium steels; and those with 0.60% to 2% carbon are high-carbon steels. Within this range, the greater the carbon content, the greater the tensile strength of the steel. The hardness of steel may be substantially increased by heating the metal until it is red hot and then quickly cooling it, a process known as quench hardening. An important component of many sxeels is cementite, a carbon-iron compound. Mild steels are ductile and are fabricated into sheets, wire, or pipe; the harder medium steels are used to make structural steel. High-carbon steels, which are extremely hard and brittle, are used in tools and cutting instruments. At carbon contents below that of steel is wrought iron, which is nearly pure iron. Because of its low carbon content (usually below 0.035%) it is forgeable and nonbrittle. Iron of high carbon content (3 to 4%), obtained when pig iron is remelted and cooled, is called cast iron. If cast iron is cooled quickly, hard but brittle white cast iron is formed; if it is cooled slowly, soft but tough gray cast iron is formed. Because it expands while cooling, cast iron is used in molds. The addition of other materials in alloys--for example, manganese or silicon--also increases the hardness of steel. The inclusion of tungsten permits high-speed drills and cutting tools to remain hard even when used at high temperatures. The inclusion of chromium and nickel improves the corrosion resistance of the steel and, within certain limits of composition, is called stainless steel. A common stainless steel contains 0.15% carbon, 18% chromium, and 8% nickel and is used in cooking utensils and food-processing equipment. The inclusion of silicon, ranging from 1 to 5%, results in an alloy that is hard and highly magnetic. An alloy with cobalt is used for permanent magnets.

LANTHANUM

Lanthanum is a chemical element, a white, malleable metal, and the first of the rere earths. Its symbol is La, its atomic number 57, and its atomic weight 138.9 Lenthanum with mass 138 is radioactive, with a half-life of 1.12×100 billion years. Lanthanum is found with other lanthanides in monazite, bastnaesite, and other minerals. It was discovered in 1839 by Swedish chemist Carl G. Mosander. Scientists have created many radioactive isotopes of lanthanum. Because lanthanum increases the refractive index of glass, it is used in manufacturing high-quality lenses. Lanthanum is also used as a reagent, as a phosphor in fluorescent lamps, and as a catalyst for cracking crude petroleum (its largest use).

LUTETIUM

Lutetium is a chemical element, a silvery white metal of the lanthanide series. Its symbol is Lu, its atomic number 71, and its atomic weight 174.97. Lutetium with mass 176 is redioactive, with a half-life of 2.2 X 10 billion years. Lutetium was discovered in 1907 by Georges Urbain, who called it Lutetia after the ancient Roman name for Paris.

MAGNESIUM

Magnesium is a silvery white metallic element of the alkaline earth metal group, which lies in group IIA of the periodic table. Its chemical symbol is Mg, atomic number 12, and atomic weight 24.312. In 1808, Sir Humphrey Davy announced that he had isolated a new element, magnesium, from the hitherto unknown magnesium oxide, which he discovered. Antoine Bussy, who is credited with discovery of the metal, isolated larger and purer amounts in 1828.

OCCURRENCE.

Magnesium is the eighth most abundant element on Earth, constituting about 2.5% of the Earth's crust. Three isotopes occur naturally: magnesium with masses of 24, 25, and 26. The most important magnesium minerals are brucite; dolomite; magnesite; and olivine. Seawater is about 0.13% magnesium and is the most important source of magnesium metal. In fresh water, dissolved magnesium and calcium salts are responsible for the hardness of water.

Production.

The primary methods of extracting magnesium are the thermal process and the electrolytic process. Approximately 20% of the magnesium produced in the world is extracted from roasted dolomite by thermal reduction. Ferrosilicon, an alloy of iron and silicon, is the reducing agent.

About 80% of the magnesium produced in the world is extracted from seawater by the electrolytic method. The seawater flows through tanks to which calcium hydroxide, has been added. The magnesium in the water is precipitated as magnesium hydroxide, and is then converted to magnesium chloride with hydrochloric acid, HCl. The magnesium chloride is dried and then electrolyzed to yield magnesium metal and chlorine gas.

Properties.

Pure magnesium is a silvery white, soft, ductile, malleable metal that oxidizes in air, producing a grayish oxide layer that protects the rest of the metal from corrosion.

Magnesium is a highly reactive metal; in compounds, it is nearly always in the +2 oxidation state. Magnesium dissolves in acids and slowly decomposes boiling water.

Uses.

Magnesium is used as a galvanic anode to prevent corrosion in pipelines, storage tanks, the hulls of ships, home water heaters, and oil tanks. Because the magnesium is dissolved before the steel in these objects is attacked, corrosion is impeded.

Finely divided magnesium burns in air with an intense white light, so the metal is used as the source of light in some flashbulbs, fireworks, and pyrotechnics. Magnesium is also used in incendiary bombs, in the production of titanium and zirconium, as a catalyst in some organic chemical reactions, and in the manufacture of copper and nickel alloys.

Magnesium has little structural strength and must be alloyed with other metals such as aluminum, zinc, or manganese when it is to be subjected to stress. In aeronautical design, the expensive metal zirconium is often the alloying additive, as it produces very strong materials. Because of their light weight, magnesium alloys are used as structural materials for the fuselages of airplanes, guided missiles, electronic equipment, portable tools, baseball catcher's masks, snowshoes, skis, boats, horseshoes, luggage, ladders, and racing cars.

Biological Significance.

Magnesium is one of the most important metals in both plants and animals. The body of an average adult contains about 25 g (0.9 oz) of magnesium; however, the specific actions of magnesium in the human body are still unknown. Magnesium is known to be an activator of many enzyme systems and acts as a depressant of the central nervous system when it is injected intravenously. For this reason, magnesium and some of its compounds are used to control convulsions resulting from tetanus and childbirth. Magnesium is found in many foods, such as meats, cereals, vegetables, and milk. The average adult ingests about 300 mg (0.01 oz) of magnesium per day. Magnesium deficiency results in weakness, dizziness, and convulsions. The kidneys regulate the amount of magnesium in the body, and magnesium overdose may result from kidney failure, hormonal disruption, or use of too much magnesium as a drug.

Magnesium Compounds.

Magnesium carbonate is a white powder that is used as a filler for paper, in cosmetics and fire-resistant and insulating materials, and for clarifying drinking water. When magnesium carbonate is boiled in water, magnesia alba is formed. Magnesia alba is used as an antacid and as a laxative.

Magnesium sulfate is marketed as epsom salts, which are used as laxatives. Magnesium sulfate is used in medicine in the treatment of arthritis and burns and as a local analgesic. It is also used for tanning leather, dyeing textiles, and in ceramics, explosives, and match manufacture. Milk of magnesia is used as an antacid and as a laxative.

A group of organic magnesium compounds, known as grignard reagents, are used in the synthesis of many organic compounds and in the production of silicones.

MANGANESE

The chemical element manganese is a silver gray metal of the transition elements. Its chemical symbol is Mn, its atomic number is 25, and its atomic weight is 54.938. Manganese was first recognized as an element in 1774 by the Swedish chemist Carl W. Scheele and isolated in the same year by his coworker, Johan G. Gahn.

ELEMENTS OF THE EARTH
AND THE HUMAN BODY

Occurrence.

The Earth's crust contains 850 ppm manganese in chemically bonded form. By far the most important manganese mineral is pyrolusite, which consists largely of manganese dioxide. Pyrolusite is brown black in color and often somewhat magnetic; the name "manganese" is a corrupted form of the Latin word for a form of magnetic stone, magnesia. Although manganese ores are not scarce, extraction is economically feasible only with open-cast mining. Extensive deposits of manganese nodules were recently discovered on the floor of the Pacific Ocean and at the bottom of several North American lakes. When large-scale mining of these nodules commences, it will be aimed primarily at the recovery of nickel, cobalt, and copper, and manganese will be a by-product.

Uses.

Pure manganese is rarely used, as it is a moderately reactive and brittle metal. About 95% of the world's annual production of manganese is used by the iron and steel industry. Manganese is added to iron because it reduces iron oxide to form manganese oxide, which dissolves well in molten slag and is easily separated from the iron. In alloys, manganese increases the durability and corrosion resistance of iron and steel and makes steel more malleable when forged. Manganese steel, or Hadfield manganese steel, contains 11-14% manganese and 1-1.5% carbon. This nonmagnetic, tough, durable, and shockproof alloy is used in grinding machinery, wrecking equipment, caterpillar trucks, and mechanical pounding equipment used in heavy-duty construction. The iron manganese alloys, which are used for making other alloys, are ferromanganese (about 80% Mn) and spiegeleisen (15-30% Mn); they contain some carbon and silicon.

Other important manganese alloys that do not contain iron include the Heusler alloys (18-25% manganese plus copper and aluminum or zinc), which are the strongest nonferrous metals; manganese copper (approximately 75% copper and 25% manganese), which has great electrical resistance; and manganin (about 83% copper, 14% manganese, and 3% nickel), which has a very slight heat-expansion coefficient and an electrical resistance nearly independent of temperature. Alloys very rich in manganese and containing nickel and copper have a high heat-expansion coefficient, however, and are used in the expanding part of bimetal thermostats.

Manganese Compounds.

The most frequently occurring valence of manganese is +2, but +4, +6, and +7 are also common, and +1, +3, and +5 are known. The doubly positive manganese ion has a light pink color in water. Two of the ion's salts, manganese chloride and manganese sulfate, are added to commercial fertilizers. The sulfate is sometimes used for making red enamel, for impregnating wood, and for staining zinc black. Manganese carbonate, yields the pigment manganese white. A number of manganese salts are used in the paint industry to accelerate the hardening of linseed oil and other drying oils.

When a manganese compound is fused with potassium nitrate, the intensely green potassium manganate is produced. By adding sulfuric acid, the intensely purple potassium permanganate is obtained. Potassium permanganate is used for bleaching and removing color from fabrics that are able to tolerate strong oxidation. In concentrated form such solutions are also used to clear clogged drain pipes.

The most important manganese compound, pyrolusite or manganese dioxide, is also an oxidizing agent. Pyrolusite is used extensively in the electrodes of dry batteries, where it absorbs liberated hydrogen gas and then chemically bonds it. It is also used as an oxygen source in fireworks and as a chemical catalyst. All other manganese compounds are made from pyrolusite.

Manganese is essential for plant growth. It is found in trace amounts in higher animals, where it activates many of the enzymes involved in metabolic processes.

Kemmer and Todd, at the University of Wisconsin, Madison, succeeded in demonstrating the essentiality of manganese in 1931. Manganese deficient animals typically exhibit retarded growth, skeletal deformities, ataxia, and convulsions. The defect in the formation of the organic bone matrix, are attributed to dysfunctions of two manganese dependent enzymes.

MOLYBDENUM

Molybdenum is a silver-white metallic chemical element of the second transition series. Its symbol is Mo; its atomic number is 42, and its atomic weight is 95.94. The name is derived from the Greek molybdos, meaning "lead." In 1778, Karl Scheele of Sweden recognized molybdenite as a distinct ore of a new element; the ore had previously been confused with graphite and lead ore. The metal was first prepared in an impure form by Hjelm in 1782. The free element does not occur in nature, but it is extracted from molybdenite, wulfenite, and powellite and is recovered as a by-product of copper and tungsten mining operations. The pure metal is prepared by the reduction of purified molybdic trioxide or ammonium molybdate with hydrogen.

Properties.

Molybdenum has a melting point of 2,617 deg C, a boiling point of 4,612 deg C, and a density of 10.22 g/cu cm. It exhibits oxidation states of 0, +1, +2, +3, +4, +5, and +6.

The metal is very hard but more ductile than the chemically similar element tungsten. Molybdenum has a high elastic modulus, and of the more readily available metals only tungsten and tantalum have higher melting points.

Uses.

Molybdenum is a valuable alloying agent, contributing to the hardenability and toughness of quenched and tempered steels. Almost all high-strength steels contain molybdenum in amounts from 0.25 to 8% by weight. Molybdenum is also used in the "hastelloys," which are nickel-based alloys with heat-resistant and corrosion-resistant properties.

Molybdenum wire is used for filaments for metal evaporation and as a filament, grid, and screen material for electronic tubes. Other applications of the metal include use as electrodes for electrically heated glass furnaces. Molybdenum sulfide is widely used as a high-temperature lubricant. The metal is also an essential trace element for plants and is important for soil fertility.

ELEMENTS OF THE EARTH
AND THE HUMAN BODY

Evidence for a physiological role for molybdenum in mammals was established after World War II through the discovery of the molybdenum-dependent enzyme, xanthine oxidase. However the nutritional molybdenum requirement of most species is so low that deficiency states cannot be readily generated in experimental animals. In chicks, a low-Mo state could eventually be induced by adding tungstsate, a molybdenum antagonist, to molybdenum-deficient diets. The Mo-deficient chicks exhibited a diminished ability to oxidize xanthine to uric acid, as expected, as dwell as increased mortality. In humans, neither molybdenum deficiency nor toxicity presently give cause for concern. However, the element was already known in the 1930s to cause a scouring disease, "teart," in cattle. Animal grazing on Mo-rich pastures develop severe diarrhea and rough, discolored coats. Since the animals rapidly lose weight, the condition is fatal unless diagnosed in time.

NEODYMIUM

Neodymium, a chemical element, is a silver white metal of the lanthanide series. Its symbol is Nd; its atomic number 60; and its atomic weight 144.24 (everage weight of its seven natural isotopes). One of its natural isotopes is radioactive. Discovered by Carl Auer von Welsbach in 1885, neodymium is used in electronics, in colored glass for astronomical lenses, and in lasers.

NICKEL

Nickel is a hard, silvery white metal, familiar from its use in coins but used mainly in alloys with other metals to improve their strength and corrosion resistance. A chemical element, nickel is a member of the transition series and belongs to group VIIIB along with iron, cobalt, palladium, platinum, and five other elements. Its chemical symbol is Ni, atomic number 28, and atomic weight 58.71.

The Earth's crust contains 0.018% nickel, although the core is believed to be much richer. Meteorites sometimes contain up to 20% nickel. Nickel was mined and used for centuries in impure form. The first fairly pure sample of nickel was prepared in 1751 by the Swedish chemist

Baron Axel F. Cronstedt from an ore German miners called Kupfernickel ("Old Nick's copper").

Pure nickel is used in electron tubes and in the galvanic (plating) industry, where many objects must be coated with nickel before they can be chrome plated. Most nickel is used in alloys where high resistance to corrosion is important, such as for chemical-reaction vessels and pump parts. Stainless steel, an alloy of iron and chromium, may contain up to 35% nickel. Special nickel alloys include alnico, cunife, and cunico, used as permanent magnets, and nichrome, which is used as electrical heating elements in many household appliances. The U.S. coin known as the "nickel" actually has 75% copper and 25% nickel.

Finely divided nickel is used as a catalyst in many reactions, such as the hydrogenation of organic compounds. It is a good catalyst for reactions with carbon monoxide because of the formation of such compounds as nickel carbonyl a rare example of a compound in which a metal has a zero valence.

In 1975, a nutritional requirement for nickel was announced by three separate research groups. In rats, inadequate dietary supply of nickel reduced growth and lowered the erythrocyte count and hemoglobin level in blood. Nickel appears to be required for proper iron utilization. However, a lack of nickel also impairs copper and zinc metabolism and lowers the activity of glucose-6-phosphate dehydrogenase and malate dehydrogenase in rat liver homoginates.

PHOSPHORUS

Phosphorus is a nonmetallic chemical element that can exist in several different allotropic forms. The chemical symbol for phosphorus is P, its atomic number is 15, and its atomic weight is 30.975. Phosphorus was first prepared by the German alchemist Hennig Brandt in 1669; in the course of his search for the philosopher's stone he obtained from a residue of evaporated urine a white solid that glowed in the dark and ignited spontaneously in air. The name phosphorus (from the Greek for "light-bringing"), which at that time was used for any substance that glows of itself, was eventually appropriated to this element. Phosphorus does not occur in elemental form in nature; it is found most commonly in apatite minerals such as fluorapatite.

Allotropes of Phosphorus.

Some ten forms of the element are known, occurring within red, white, and black (violet) phosphorus categories or as mixtures of them. White phosphorus consists of molecular P and can exist in an alpha form, which is stable at room temperature, and a beta form, stable below -78 deg C (-108 deg F). White phosphorus is a waxlike substance, very toxic and extremely flammable. When it is exposed to air in the dark, it emits a greenish light and gives off white fumes. It can ignite spontaneously. White phosphorus is used in incendiary and napalm bombs and in rat poison.

Red phosphorus, a more stable form than white, can be obtained by heating white phosphorus to 250 deg C in a closed vessel. Red phosphorus is often considered a mixture of white and black phosphorus. It neither phosphoresces nor spontaneously burns in air. It is used in industry as part of the coating of safety matches and in the manufacture of tracer bullets, smoke screens, and skywriting compounds.

Upon heating to temperatures near 300 deg C (570 deg F) for several days, red phosphorus is converted to black phosphorus, a much less common form. Black phosphorus is flaky, like graphite, and has some metallic properties. It is the least reactive of the forms.

Phosphates.

Nearly all the phosphorus used in commerce is in the form of phosphates, the salts derived from phosphoric acid. Large amounts of phosphate-containing fertilizer are used to enhance soil fertility. Sodium triphosphate is used in detergents because it softens water and disperses inorganic soiling substances. A serious disadvantage of using phosphates in detergents, however, is the fact that the phosphates later end up in natural bodies of water, where they act as fertilizers, causing algae in the water to proliferate. Phosphates are also used in toothpastes and as polishing agents. Monocalcium phosphate and sodium acid pyrophosphate are leavening agents used in baking powder.

Biological Role of Phosphorus.

Phosphorus, exclusively in the form of phosphates, is found in all forms of life. Phosphates are essential to the energy-transfer reactions necessary to sustain life processes. Of major importance is adenosine triphosphate (ATP), which is involved in nearly every metabolic or photosynthetic reaction. Reactions that are not spontaneous themselves are driven by the chemical energy released when a high-energy phosphate group is released from ATP. The resultant adenosine diphosphate (ADP) reforms to ATP for further participation in reactions.

Phosphates are also important ingredients of bone; the human skeleton contains about 1.4 kg (about 3 lb) of phosphates as calcium phosphate. Phosphates also form part of a number of coenzymes and the parts of the nucleic acids that comprise chromosomes.

POTASSIUM

The chemical element potassium is a soft, light, silver white metal. It is a member of the alkali metals, a group (IA of the periodic table) of elements with similar physical and chemical properties. Its chemical symbol is K (from kalium, the Latinized version of the Arabic word for "alkali"); its atomic number, 19; and atomic weight, 39.098.

Potash, or potassium carbonate, was well known and had important industrial uses in glass manufacture well before 1700; however, it was often mistaken for sodium carbonate and only their decidedly different sources prevented total confusion. Sodium carbonate (soda) is most often found as a mineral; potash was originally derived from the ashes of vegetable materials. Even before the discovery and differentiation of their cationic elements, potash and sodium carbonate could be identified by their crystal structures. On Oct. 6, 1807, Sir Humphry Davy connected a piece of solid potash to the poles of a battery and caused the release of a new metal at the negative pole. He named it potassium, from potash, and within a short time had determined many of its physical and chemical properties.

ELEMENTS OF THE EARTH
AND THE HUMAN BODY

Occurrence.

In cosmic abundance potassium is the 20th most common element; in solar abundance, 17th; and in the Earth's crust, 7th. About 2.6% of the Earth's crust consists of potassium. It is far too reactive to exist in the free state and thus occurs combined as compounds such as carnallite, orthoclase feldspar, leucite, potash mica, and kaolin. Seawater contains about 0.4 kg (1 lb) potassium oxide per cu m, about 70% of which is readily recoverable. Commercial quantities of the oxide are found in Searle's Lake, Calif.; Carlsbad, N.Mex.; Stassfurt, East Germany; Mulhouse, France; Cardona, Spain; the Dead Sea; Kalusz, Poland; and Saskatchewan, Canada. Potassium can be recovered from the ashes of plants, which remove it from the soil.

Chemical Properties.

Potassium is an alkali metal. These metals, family IA of the periodic table, are the most reactive ones. In general, chemical reactivity within the family increases from the small atoms at the top of the table to the large at the bottom, so potassium is more active than lithium and sodium and less active than rubidium and cesium.

Potassium readily reacts with the halogens to form potassium halides and with oxygen to form potassium oxide and potassium peroxide. Because of their electron arrangement and relatively large size and small charge, potassium atoms are not conducive to complex ion formation or ion formation by any but ionic bonds.

Potassium reacts with sodium to form an intermetallic compound. It reacts violently with water and explosively both with acids and with liquid bromine, and forms an explosive carbonyl. An intimate mixture of 75% potassium nitrate, 15% carbon (charcoal), and 10% sulfur is the "black powder" used as gunpowder for more than 2,200 years.

Production. Except for its greater reactivity, potassium is similar to sodium. It can be produced by electrolytic reduction of fused potassium hydroxide (KOH) or fused potassium chloride (KCl). Although this method of production is occasionally used to make laboratory quantities of the metal, the energy requirements are too great for commercial use.

Other laboratory methods of manufacturing potassium include electrolysis of fused potassium cyanide (KCN), by heating potassium chloride (KCl) with metallic calcium in a vacuum and distilling the potassium as it is formed, or by heating potassium hydroxide (KOH) with iron, aluminum, or magnesium.

Commercial uses of potassium are most often also satisfied by the more easily recovered sodium. Therefore only modest amounts of the former metal are produced. One industrial method of production uses sodium vapor to reduce molten potassium chloride at 880 deg C. The potassium vapor formed is drawn off and condensed to liquid metal.

Important Compounds and Uses.

When dispersed on supports of carbon or potassium carbonate, metallic potassium is used as a catalyst for various reactions such as the dimerization of propene to 4-methyl-1-pentene. Dissolved in mercury to form an amalgam, potassium metal yields a liquid reducing agent. Dissolved in alcohols it gives alkoxides, which are reducing agents and also a source of nucleophilic ions. Potassium alkyls can be used for metallation reactions and when dispersed on an inert support may act as a catalyst in the polymerization or isomerization of alkenes.

Because potassium is vital to plant growth, large quantities are annually used in the form of potassium nitrate. Until World War I the United States imported most of its potassium nitrate from the mines in the prehistoric seabeds of Europe. When these sources became unavailable during the war, the brines of Searles Lake, Calif., became the principal source of this chemical. Until the improvement (1919) of equipment and methods, however, separation methods were inefficient.

Potassium phosphate is also an important potassium salt. For many years large quantities of potassium phosphate have been used as "builders" in enhancing surfactant performance of detergents. This use is now decreasing in response to the need to remove phosphates from the environment.

Potassium carbonate is a third important potassium compound. It is prepared by the Leblanc process from potassium chloride and magnesium carbonate. Its principal use is in the manufacture of glass.

ELEMENTS OF THE EARTH
AND THE HUMAN BODY

Although most alkali metal compounds are appreciably soluble, a few are not and may be used for separation, isolation, and identification of the metals. The common sparingly soluble compounds of potassium are: potassium fluorosilicate, potassium chloroplatinate, potassium perchlorate, and potassium sodium cobaltinitrite.

PRASEODYMIUM

Praseodymium is a chemical element, a silvery white metal of the lanthanide series. Its symbol is Pr, its atomic number 59, and its atomic weight 140. Pure praseodymium was first obtained in 1885 by C. A. von Welsbach. The name is derived from the Greek for "leekgreen," referring to the color of the element's salts. Praseodymium salts are used to color glass and ceramic glazes, and its oxide is used, along with other rare-earth metal oxides, as a core material for carbon arcs.

RUBIDIUM

Rubidium is a silvery white radioactive chemical element and a member of the alkali metals, a group that includes sodium, potassium, and cesium. Its symbol is Rb; its atomic number, 37; and its atomic weight, 85.4678. Its name is derived from the Latin rubidius, meaning "deepest red." Rubidium is relatively abundant and is considered to rank 16th in the Earth's crust. It was discovered in 1861 by Robert Bunsen and Gustav Kirchhoff in a spectroscopic examination of the mineral lepidolite. The pure metal is usually prepared by reducing the chloride with calcium. Like other members of the alkali metal group, rubidium ignites spontaneously in air and reacts violently with water, setting fire to the liberated hydrogen. The refined metal must consequently be kept under dry mineral oil, in a vacuum, or in an inert atmosphere.

Rubidium is a soft metal that can be liquid at room temperature, although the pure element melts at 38.89 deg C (102 deg F) and boils at 688 deg C (1,270 deg F). Of the 17 known isotopes of rubidium, only Rb-85 and Rb-87 occur naturally. Rubidium-87 is a beta emitter with a half-life of $5 \times 10(11)$ years.

Rubidium has oxidation states of +1, +2, +3, and +4. It is one of the most reactive metals, resembling potassium in its chemical properties. A compound of rubidium has the highest room-temperature conductivity of any known ionic crystal. The element is used as a getter in vacuum tubes, as a component in photocells, and in the making of special glasses.

SAMARIUM

Samarium is a chemical element, a very hard, silvery white metal of the lanthanide series. Its symbol is Sm; its atomic number, 62; and its atomic weight, 150.4 (average weight of its seven natural isotopes). Three natural samarium isotopes are radioactive: Sm = 147, Sm = 148, and Sm = 149. Samarium was discovered in 1879 by Lecoq de Boisbaudran, who isolated it from samarskite. The metal ignites in air at 150 deg C (302 deg F). Because one of its isotopes has a high cross section of neutron absorption, samarium is used in the control rods of nuclear reactors. An alloy of samarium with cobalt is used to make a magnetic material with the highest resistance to demagnetization of any known material.

SCANDIUM

Scandium is a silvery white metallic chemical element, the first member of the first transition series. Its symbol is Sc; its atomic number, 21; and its atomic weight, 44.9559. The name is derived from Scandinavia, where the element was discovered in the minerals euxenite and gadolinite. In 1876, L. F. Nilson prepared about 2 g of high purity scandium oxide. It was subsequently established that scandium corresponds to the element "ekaboron" predicted by Mendeleyev on the basis of a gap in the periodic table.

Scandium occurs in small quantities in more than 800 minerals and causes the blue color of aquamarine beryl. It is a relatively soft and light metal with a melting point of 1,541 deg C, a boiling point of 2831 deg C, and a density of 2.989 g/cu cm. The chemical properties of scandium resemble those of yttrium and the rare earth metals rather than those of aluminum or titanium. It has 11 known isotopes. Unlike other transition metals, scandium exhibits an oxidation state of exclusively +3. At present scandium has no commercial uses.

SELENIUM

Selenium is the third member of the chalogen group (VIA) of elements of the periodic table, coming after oxygen and sulfur and preceding tellurium. Its chemical symbol is Se, atomic number 34, and atomic weight 78.96. Its name is derived from the Greek selene, meaning Moon. It was discovered in 1817 by Jons Jacob Berzelius in association with tellurium.

Selenium is present in some rare minerals, such as crookesite and clausthalite, and in some sulfur deposits and sulfide ores. It is a rare element forming only 9 X 10 to the power of - 6% of the Earth's crust. Selenium exists in at least three allotropic forms: amorphous selenium is either red in powder form or black in vitreous form; crystalline monoclinic selenium is deep red; and crystalline hexagonal selenium, the most stable form, is a metallic gray. Natural selenium (gray) consists of six stable isotopes and has a melting point of 217 deg C, a boiling point of 684.9 deg C, and a specific gravity of 4.79. The most important oxidation states are +4 and +6.

The chemical reactions of selenium resemble those of sulfur and are typically nonmetallic in nature. In progressing through the chalcogen group of elements there is a striking decrease in oxidizing properties, and the hydrides hydrogen selenide and hydrogen teleride are better reducing agents than hydrogen. Selenium reacts directly with many metals although not with the noble metals. Hydrogen selenide, may be prepared by the direct combination of the elements but is better prepared by the action of dilute hydrochloric acid on a selenide. Selenium reacts less readily with oxygen to form the dioxide than does sulfur. The flourides, may be prepared by direct reaction of selenium with fluorine. Selenious acid, is formed when the soluble selenium dioxide, is dissolved in water. Selenium dioxide is a good oxidizing agent and is used in certain organic syntheses. Selenic acid, which has similar properties to sulfuric acid, is formed by dissolving selenium trioxide, in water.

ELEMENTS OF THE EARTH
AND THE HUMAN BODY

The principal commercial source of selenium is in the anode sludge obtained from the electrolytic refining of copper. Selenium is recovered by roasting the sludges with soda or sulfuric acid. Elemental selenium is claimed to be practically nontoxic, but hydrogen selenide and other selenium compounds are extremely toxic, resembling arsenic in their physiological behavior.

Selenium exhibits both photovoltaic action, whereby light is converted directly into electricity; and photoconductive activity, whereby electrical resistance is decreased with increased light exposure. As a consequence, selenium is used in the production of photocells, exposure meters, and solar cells. Selenium also finds extensive application in rectifiers, a result of its ability to convert alternating electric current to direct current. Selenium behaves as a p-type semiconductor and is being increasingly used in electronic and solid-state devices. Other applications of the element include its use in the glass industry to decolorize glass, as a photographic toner, as an additive in steel production, and in xerographic reproduction.

Long known and feared only as a severe poison, selenium was shown in 1957 to be the integral part of a powerfully antihepatonecrotic factor isolated from pork kidney, and thus became a nutritionally essential element. (Schwartz and Foltz, 1957)

In 1957, exudative diathesis in chicks was shown to be a selenium deficiency disease. After annually causing millions of dollars of damage to the poultry industry, exudative diathesis became readily preventable through the addition of 0.1 ppm if selenium to the feed. Identification of "white muscle disease," a muscular dystrophy in lambs and calves of New Zealand and Oregon, was similarly shown to be caused by selenium deficiency (Muth et al., 1958).

Selenium was shown in 1972 to be the functional component of the enzyme glutathine peroxidase (Rotruck et al., 1972. The enzyme assures the maintenance of the structural integrity of liver and other cell membranes by protecting them from the destructive effects of oxygen radicals. Oxygen radicals are formed during lipid metabolism, but also on exposure of organs and tissues to ionizing radiation, as well as by certain drugs. Selenium in required for the maintenance of fertility, the functioning of the eye, the heart, and the immune system. It also exerts protective effects against certain heavy metals, notably mercury and cadmium. It has also been identified as a nutritional cancer prevention agent. An inflammatory, painful disease related to arthritis, which is locally known as "big joint disease," is also probably caused by selenium deficiency and/or molybdenum deficiency. (Zhu, 1980).

SILICON

The element silicon is a dark-colored crystalline semimetal in the same periodic table group as carbon and germanium. The name silicon is derived from the Latin silex or silicis, meaning flint. Its symbol is Si, atomic number 14, and atomic weight 28.0855. In 1811, Joseph Gay-Lussac and Baron Louis Thenard probably prepared impure amorphous silicon by reacting potassium with silicon tetrafluoride. The credit for discovering the element is usually given to Jons Jacob Berzelius, who also prepared amorphous silicon in 1824 by the same method but purified the product by repeated washings that removed fluorosilicates.

Silicon is present in the Sun and stars and is a major constituent of the class of meteorites known as aerolites. It is present in the Earth's crust to the extent of 25.7% and is the second most abundant element, next to oxygen. The free element silicon is not found in nature, but it occurs either as the oxide silica, in such forms as sand, quartz, and rock crystal, or as silicates in such minerals as granite, asbestos, clay, and mica. Silicon has a melting point of 1,410 deg C, a boiling point of 2,355 deg C, a density of 2.33 g/cu cm at 25 deg C, and a valence of 4. It is a relatively inert element but is attacked by halogens and dilute alkali.

An important class of silicon-containing compounds is silicones, which are prepared from organosilicon chlorides such as dimethylsilyl chloride. Hydrolysis followed by condensation yields macromolecular structures. The silicon polymers, which range from liquids to hard solids, have useful water-repellent and temperature-resistant properties. Silicone rubbers retain their elasticity at much lower temperatures than ordinary rubber.

Silicon is prepared commercially by heating silica and carbon in an electric furnace with carbon electrodes. Silicon is an important constituent in several structural materials; in the form of sand and clay it is used to make concrete and brick, and sand is also the principal component of glass. Carborundum (silicon carbide) is one of the most widely used abrasives for cutting and grinding metals. Silicon is important in plant and animal life; diatoms extract silica from water to build up their cell walls, and silica is present in the ashes of plants and in human skeletons.

The second most abundant element in the lithosphere, silicon is nevertheless a biological "trace" element, for only traces of it are needed and taken up by mammals. Silicon-deficient rats showed impaired growth, a disturbance of bone formation and was particularly noticeable in the skull, and a diminution in the pigmentation of the incisors.

STRONTIUM

Strontium is a soft, silvery metal with physical and chemical properties similar to those of calcium. Its symbol is Sr; its atomic number, 38; and its atomic weight, 87.62. First isolated (1808) by Sir Humphry Davy, strontium is found in the minerals strontianite and celestite. Many radioactive isotopes of strontium are produced in nuclear reactors. Strontium 90, with a half-life of 28 years, is formed in nuclear explosions; because it accumulates in the bones, it is considered the most dangerous component of radioactive fallout. Strontium salts impart red color to flames and are used in red signal flares, fireworks, and tracer bullets.

TERBIUM

Terbium is a chemical element, a very rare silver-gray metal of the lanthanide series. Its symbol is Tb, its atomic number 65, and its atomic weight 158.9254. Terbium was discovered in 1843 by C. G. Mosander; it was first extracted in fairly pure form by G. Urbain in 1905. It is not used in industry but is studied because of its complex magnetic behavior.

ELEMENTS OF THE EARTH
AND THE HUMAN BODY

TIN

Tin, a solid, rather unreactive metal, in group IVA of the periodic table, has an atomic number of 50 and an atomic weight of 118.69. Its chemical symbol, Sn, is derived from stannum, the Latin word for tin. Tin has ten naturally occurring isotopes; the most abundant is one having a mass of 120 (32.85%). Bronze, an alloy of copper and tin, has been known since 2500-2000 BC. The first inclusion of tin in bronze was probably an accidental result of tin ore being found in copper ore; pure tin was probably obtained at a later date.

Tin is relatively rare (about 0.001% in the Earth's crust) and is obtained from its chief ore, cassiterite ($SnO(2)$), a naturally occurring tin oxide, by various refining methods, including carbon reduction. Important ore deposits are found in Malaysia, Indonesia, Zaire, Nigeria, and Bolivia.

Physical Properties

White tin, the element's familiar allotropic form, is a silvery white, soft, ductile metal that melts at 232 deg C and boils at 2,270 deg C. Below 13.2 deg C (55.8 deg F), pure metallic tin slowly converts to gray tin, a different crystalline form that is less dense and lacks the metallic properties of white tin. The white form is normally used; gray tin has few, if any, uses.

Chemical Properties

In its chemical compounds, tin exhibits two common oxidation states, +2 and +4. Tin dissolves in hydrochloric acid, reacting to yield stannous chloride ($SnCh(2)$), and hydrogen gas. Concentrated nitric acid oxidizes tin to the +4 oxidation state, forming stannic oxide, $SnO(2)$. A strong base, such as sodium hydroxide, dissolves tin to form a stannate, a chemical salt.

When exposed to the atmosphere and moisture, tin forms a protective oxide coating that resists further corrosion. When tin reacts with excess chlorine gas, stannous chloride, $SnCl(2)$, a colorless liquid and electrical conductor, is formed. The reaction of tin with hydroflyoric acid yields stannous fluoride, $SnF(2)$, a white, water-soluble compound that is added to toothpaste to help prevent tooth decay.

Alloys

Tin is a major component in many useful alloys. When mixed with tin to form bronze, copper is easier to cast and has superior mechanical properties. Pewter is an alloy of tin hardened with antimony and copper. Tin alloys are also used in solder, bearings, and type metals. Commonly used solders are alloys of tin and lead.

In 1970, Schwarz et al. reported the first positive growth responses of tin in young rats at levels from 0.5 to 2 ppm in the diet. It is possible that tin, by virtue of its existence in the oxidation states and its ability to form complexes with a variety of chemicals, acts as an electron transfer catalyst. however, more work is required to establish its essentiality and nurtitional roles.

TITANIUM

Titanium is a silvery gray metal resembling polished steel. A transition element, its symbol is Ti, its atomic number 22, and its atomic weight 47.90. Titanium was first discovered as its oxygen compound in 1791 by William Gregor and named in 1795 by Martin H. Klaproth after the Titans, the giants of Greek mythology. Nevertheless, the pure metal was not obtained until 1910 and remained a laboratory curiosity until an economical purification process was discovered in 1946.

Occurrence.

Titanium is the ninth most abundant element, comprising about 0.63% of the Earth's crust. Analyses of rock samples from the Moon indicate titanium is far more abundant there; some rocks consisted of 12% titanium by weight. The most important titanium minerals are anatase, brookite, and rutile, all forms of titanium dioxide.

Uses.

Because titanium is as strong as steel and 45% lighter, it is especially suitable for use in aviation and astronautics. About 50% of titanium production is used for jet engine components (rotors, fins, and compressor parts). Titanium alloys readily with other metals such as aluminum and tin. The alloy composition Ti + 2.5% tin + 5% aluminum is used when high strength at high temperatures is required; and the alloy Ti + 8% aluminum + molybdenum + vanadium is used in applications at low temperatures. Each supersonic transport (SST) contains about 270,000 kg (600,000 lb) of titanium.

Compounds.

Not many titanium compounds are used commercially. Titanium tetrachloride is a colorless liquid that fumes in moist air; it is used in the manufacture of artificial pearls and iridescent glass and, by the military, to create smokescreens. The most important titanium oxide is titanium dioxide, which is a white substance with a high reflective power. It is used extensively in both house paint and artist's paint, replacing the poisonous lead white. Titanium dioxide is processed at very high temperatures into artificial rutile, which is used as a semiprecious stone (titania). Titania has a light yellow color and a higher index of refraction than diamond but is rather soft.

VANADIUM

Vanadium is a bright white metallic chemical element of the first series of transition metals. It has the symbol V; its atomic number is 23, and its atomic weight is 50.9414. The element was discovered in 1801 by Andres M. del Rio, but at the time the finding was dismissed as impure chromium. The element was rediscovered in 1830 by Nils G. Sefstrom, who named it in honor of the Scandinavian goddess Vanadis.

Among the 65 or so minerals in which vanadium occurs, the more important sources of the metal include carnotite, patronite, roscoelite, and vanadinite. Other sources of vanadium are in phosphate rock, certain iron ores, and some crude oils in the form of organic complexes. The extraction of vanadium from petroleum ash is a possible future source of the element. High-purity vanadium is obtained by reduction of vanadium trichloride with magnesium or with magnesium-sodium mixtures. Because the major use of the metal is as an alloying agent for steel, pure vanadium is seldom extracted, and the bulk of the metal is currently made by the reduction of vanadium pentoxide with calcium.

Natural vanadium consists of two isotopes, V-50 and V-51, the former being slightly radioactive with a half-life of 6 X 10 to the 15th power years. Seven other radioisotopes of the element have been synthesized. The pure metal is soft and ductile, with a melting point of 1,890 deg C, a boiling point of 3,380 deg C, and a density of 6.11 g/cu cm. The outer electronic configuration of vanadium exhibits oxidation states of -1, 0, +1, +2, +3, +4, and +5 in a wide variety of complex ions and coordination complexes.

Vanadium is resistant to corrosion by alkali, sulfuric and hydrochloric acids, and salt water but oxidizes rapidly above about 660 deg C. Because the metal has good structural strength and a low fission neutron cross-section, it finds extensive application in the nuclear industry. The metal is also used in forming rust-resistant spring and high-speed tool steels; about 80% of the production of vanadium is used to make ferrovanadium or as a steel additive. Vanadium pentoxide is used in ceramics and as a catalyst. Vanadium and its compounds are toxic.

Vanadium stimulated the pigmentation of incisors in rats at .05 to .1 ppm. It was also demonstrates that vanadium-deficient chicks and rats develop higher plasma cholesterol levels than the controls. Vanadium appears to act as a biocatalyst of oxidation of certain substrates. It is possible that this explains its cholesterol-lowering effect in humans.

YTTERBIUM

Ytterbium is a silvery, soft metal, an element of the lanthanide series group IIIB. Its chemical symbol is Yb; its atomic number, 70; and atomic weight, 173.04. Seven isotopes exist in nature. Ytterbium is difficult to separate from the other rare-earth elements with which it is found. It was discovered (1878) by Jean C. G. de Marignac, who named it for a Swedish town, Ytterby. Few commercial uses exist.

YTTRIUM

Yttrium is one of four chemical elements (the others being erbium, terbium, and ytterbium) named after Ytterby, a village in Sweden rich in unusual minerals and rare earths. Yttrium is a metal with a silvery luster and properties closely resembling those of rare-earth metals; for this reason it is frequently classified with the elements of the lanthanice series. Its symbol is Y; its atomic number, 39; and atomic weight, 88.9059. Its principal use is as the matrix of europium-activated red phosphors that give the red color in color television tubes.

ZINC

Zinc is a metal of major importance in the modern world. It is widely used as a coating to protect iron and steel from corrosion and as a component of useful alloys. The symbol for zinc is Zn, its atomic number is 30, and its atomic weight is 65.37. The name of the element derives from the German word for the metal, zink, but the origin is unknown.

Zinc metal was first produced in India and China during the Middle Ages. The ancient Egyptians used brass, but the alloy was made by smelting copper ore that already contained zinc. The Romans made brass by fusing zinc oxide or carbonate minerals with copper metal. The extraction and production of metallic zinc did not start in Europe until the 1740s.

Occurrence.

Zinc, the 25th most abundant element, is widely distributed in nature, making up between 0.0005% and 0.02% of the Earth's crust. The most abundant and important zinc minerals are the sulfide (sphalerite or zinc blende), the carbonate (smithsonite), the silicate (calamine), and a mixed oxide with manganese and iron (franklinite). The sulfide and carbonate are the principal sources of the metal.

Physical Properties.

Zinc metal normally appears dull gray because of an oxide or basic carbonate coating, but when freshly polished it is bluish white and lustrous. It is moderately hard, brittle at room temperature, and a good conductor of electricity. The melting point of pure zinc (419.5 deg C) is a reference point adopted by the U.S. National Bureau of Standards for the International Practical Temperature Scale. The boiling point (907 deg C) is sufficiently low to permit practical purification by distillation in the pyrometallurgical process.

Chemical Properties.

Zinc belongs to group IIB in the periodic table. The metal is a good reducing agent and is used as such in many laboratory applications. Zinc dissolves in aqueous acids or bases, forming hydrogen gas and zinc ion or zincate ion, respectively. Zinc forms compounds only in the +2 oxidation state.

Uses.

The two major uses of zinc metal are (1) to coat iron and steel--a process called galvanizing--to prevent corrosion and (2) as a component of several alloys. An additional 5% to 10% of total zinc production goes into dry-cell battery cans and sheet zinc for photoengraving. Zinc protects iron from rusting because it is the stronger reducing agent of the two metals. As long as physical contact is maintained, zinc will be preferentially oxidized; the iron merely acts as an electrical conductor to transfer electrons from zinc to oxygen. The best-known zinc alloy is brass, which is made of copper with 3% to 45% zinc. Die-casting alloys (96% zinc, 4% aluminum, trace magnesium) account for 25% of the zinc produced and are used to make accurately formed metal components by injection molding.

The most widely used zinc compounds are the oxide, the sulfide, and the chloride. The oxide is used as a reinforcer in rubber tires, a white paint pigment, a ceramic glaze, and an opaque base in cosmetics, salves, and lotions. The sulfide is used as a phosphor in fluorescent lamps and cathode ray tubes and as a white pigment. The chloride is useful as a soldering flux, a dry-cell battery electrolyte, and a wood preservative.

Zinc is of very low toxicity in its ordinary compounds and is an essential trace element in plant and animal life. A zinc deficiency in the human diet retards growth and maturity and produces anemia.

Three years after the discovery of the essentiality of manganese, the Wisconsin group demonstrated that zinc was also an essential element in mammals, but it took another 22 years until zinc deficiency was shown to be responsible for Laennec's cirrhosis, a type of cirrhosis formerly thought to be due to alcoholism. The accelerating effects of zinc on wound healing were objectively described only less than thirty years ago. Zinc is required by nearly 100 different mammalian enzymes. It is essential for the maintenance of growth, development, cell division, protein, and DNA synthesis. In spite of its central importance, its roles in human and animal nutrition are only now beginning to be recognized. Nutritional zinc deficiency causes dwarfism and hypogonadism in boys in Iran and Egypt. Marginal zinc deficiency produces a variety of mild or vague symptoms, including inappetence, smell and taste dysfunctions. These have since been shown to occur in a surprisingly high percentage of American adults.

Bibilography

Alexander, W., & Street, A., Metals in the Service of Man (1972)

Anfinsen, C. B., *Aspects of Protein Synthesis* (1970)

Avers, Charlotte T., *Cell Biology* (1976)

Aylett, B. J., *The Chemistry of Zinc, Cadmium and Mercury* (1975)

Babkin, B. P., Secretory Mechanisms of the Digestive Glands, 2d ed. (1950)

Bailar, J. C., Jr., ed., The Chemistry of the Coordination Compounds (1956)

Baldwin, William L., *The World Tin Market: Political Pricing and Economic Competition* (1983)

Barrett, Graham, ed., Chemistry and Biochemistry of the Amino Acids (1985)

Barry, B. T., and Thwaites, C. G., *Tin and Its Alloys and Compounds* (1983)

Beaton, G. H., and Bengoa, J. M., eds., Nutrition in Preventative Medicine (1976)

Berger, Melvin, *Enzymes in Action* (1971)

Block, Zenas, *It's All on the Label: Understanding Food, Additives, and Nutrition* (1981)

Bourne, G. H., and Kidder, G. W., eds., Biochemistry and Physiology of Nutrition, 2 vols. (1953)

Boyer, P.D., ed., The Enzymes (1970)

Briggs, M. H., Vitamins in Human Biology and Medicine (1981)

Butts, Allison, Silver: Economics, Metallurgy, and Use (1967, repr. 1975)

Calder, Nigel, *The Life Game: Evolution and the New Biology* (1974)

Calvin, Melvin, *Chemical Evolution* (1969)

Chaney, Margaret S., and Ross, Margaret L., Nutrition, 9th ed. (1979)

Clark, R., and Brown, D., *The Chemistry of Vanadium, Niobium, and Tantalum* (1975).

Consumer Guide, The Vitamin Book (1979)

Corbridge, D., Phosphorus (1978)

Cotton, F. A., and Wilkinson, G., Advanced Inorganic Chemistry, 3d ed. (1972)

Cotton, F. A., and Wilkinson, G., Basic Inorganic Chemistry (1976)

Crook, Henry M.D. *Use of Colloids in Health & Disease*, Becker, Robert O., M.D., The Body Electric, (1985)

Curtin, Sharon, *Nobody Ever Died of Old Age* (1973)

Czerny, Peter G., The Great Great Salt Lake (1976)

Davenport, Horace W., Physiology of the Digestive Tract, 4th ed. (1977)

Dyke, S. F., The Chemistry of the Vitamins (1965)

Ebsworth, E. A. V., *Volatile Silicon Compounds* (1963)

Bibliography

Ebsworth, E. A. V., *Volatile Silicon Compounds* (1963)

Emmelin, N. G., The Physiology of the Salivary Glands (1961)

Emsley, John, *The Chemistry of Phosphorus* (1976)

Engel, Leonard, *The New Genetics* (1967)

Farley, John, *The Spontaneous Generation Controversy from Descartes to Oparin* (1979)

Folsome, Clair E., ed., *Origin of Life: Readings from "Scientific American"* (1978);

Fox, Sidney W., and Dose, Klaus, Molecular Evolution and the Origins of Life, 2d ed. (1977)

Frolkis, V. V., *Aging and Life-Prolonging Processes* (1982)

Fruton, J. S., *Molecules and Life* (1972)

Furia, Thomas E., ed., Handbook of Food Additives (1979)

Gortner, Willis A., and Freydberg, Nicholas, The Food Additives Book (1982)

Groseclose, E. E., The Silken Metal: Silver, Past, Present, Prospective (1975)

Haberecht, R. R., and Kern, E. L., *Semiconductor Silicon* (1969)

Hager, Thomas, and Kessler, Lauren, *Staying Young: The Whole Truth About Aging, and What You Can Do To Slow Its Progress* (1987)

Hampel, C. A., ed., The Encyclopedia of the Chemical Elements (1968)

Harvey, Hildebrande W., The Chemistry and Fertility of Sea Waters, 2d ed. (1957)

Hochschild, Arlie Russell, *The Unexpected Community* (1978)

Howe, P. S., Basic Nutrition in Health and Disease, 5th ed. (1971)

Hoyle, Fred, and Wickramsinghe, N. C., *Lifecloud: The Origin of Life in the Universe* (1979)

Hughes, Christopher C., The Additives Guide (1987)

Hunter, Beatrice T., The Additives Book, rev. ed. (1980)

Igoe, Robert S., Dictionary of Food Ingredients (1983)

Jacobson, Michael F., Eater's Digest: The Consumer's Factbook of Food Additives (1982)

Johnson, J. C., ed., Food Additives: Recent Developments (1983)

Johnson, Leonard R., *Gastrointestinal Physiology* (1977)

Jones, F. A., et al., Clinical Gastroenterology, 2d ed. (1968)

Kalish, Richard A., *The Later Years* (1977)

Karnola, Josepha M., *Food Additives* (1984)

King, Ethel M., *The Fountain of Youth and Juan Ponce de Leon* (1963)

Krause, M. V., and Hunschler, M. A., Food Nutrition and Diet Therapy, 5th ed. (1972)

Kudryavtsev, A. A., The Chemistry and Technology of Selenium and Tellurium, 2d ed., trans. by E. M. Elkin (1974)

Kudryavtsev, A. A., The Chemistry and Technology of Selenium and Tellurium, 2d ed., trans. by E. M. Elkin (1974)

Kutsky, R. J., Handbook of Vitamins, Minerals and Hormones, 2d ed. (1981)

Bibliography

Kutsky, Roman J. Ph.D., Van Nostrand Reinhold Company, Handbook of Vitamins, Minerals and Hormones 2nd ed. (1981)

Latour, John Paul, The ABCs of Vitamins, Minerals, and Natural Foods (1972)

Lehninger, A. L., Biochemistry, 2d ed. (1975)

Lesser, Michael, *Nutrition and Vitamin Therapy* (1979)

Levine, Louis, Biology of the Gene, 2d ed. (1973)

Levy, Joseph V., Vitamins; Their Use and Abuse (1976)

Lewis, C. M., Basic and Family Nutrition, 2d ed. (1984)

Long, Charles H., Alpha: *The Myths of Creation* (1963)

Marquand, Josephine, *Life: Its Nature, Origins, and Distribution* (1971)

Massey, A. G., et al., *The Chemistry of Copper, Silver, and Gold* (1975)

Mathewson, C. H., ed., *Zinc: The Science and Technology of the Metal, Its Alloys and Compounds* (1959; repr. 1970)

Mendeloff, Albert, and Dunn, James P., *Digestive Diseases* (1971)

Metzler, David E., Biochemistry (1977)

Milne, Lorus and Margery, *The Ages of Life* (1968)

Moore, Ruth, *The Coil of Life: The Story of the Great Discoveries in the Life Sciences* (1961)

Morton, J. E., Guts: The Form and Function of the Digestive System (1967)

Moss, D. W., *Enzymes* (1968)

Nebergall, William H., et al., General Chemistry, 5th ed. (1976)

Nicholls, D., The Chemistry of Iron, Cobalt and Nickel (1975)

Nicolls, D., *The Chemistry of Iron, Cobalt and Nickel* (1975).

O'Donnell, T. A., *The Chemistry of Fluorine* (1975)

Oparin, Aleksandr I., *Genesis and Evolutionary Development of Life* (1968)

Passwater, Richard, A Beginner's Introduction to Vitamins (1983)

Pattison, E. Mansell, *The Experience of Dying* (1977);

Price, Raye C., Barrier of Salt: The Story of the Great Salt Lake, 2d ed. (1976)

Rahn, A., *Tin in Organic Synthesis* (1987)

Rennert, O. M., and Chan, Waiyee, eds., Metabolism of Trace Minerals in Man, 2 vols. (1984)

Rollinson, C. L., The Chemistry of Chromium, Molybdenum and Tungsten (1975)

Rosenfeld, Irene, and Beath, O. A., Selenium, 2d ed. (1964)

Ryall, R. J., The Digestive System (1976)

Saunders, Barbara, *Understanding Additives* (1988)

Schwarz, K. (1977): Clinical Chemistry and Chemical Toxicology, ed S.S. Brown. Amsterdam

Sleisinger, Marvin, and Fortram, John, *Gastrointestinal Disease* (1973)

Smith, Ivan C., and Carson, Bonnie L., Silver, vol. 2 (1977)

Bibliography

Solomons, N. W., and Rosenberg, I. H., Absorption and Metabolism of Mineral Nutrients (1984)

Sverdrup, Harald U., et al., The Oceans: Their Physics, Chemistry and General Biology (1942)

Swaminathan, M. and & Bhagwan,R. K. (1969): Minerals in our Food, 6th edn p 31 Madras: Ganesh & Co.

Toy, Arthur D., *Phosphorus Chemistry in Everyday Living* (1976)

Tribe, M. A., et al., *Protein Synthesis* (1976)

Trotman-Dickenson, A. F., ed., Comprehensive Inorganic Chemistry, vol. 4 (1973)

Turekian, Karl K., Oceans, 2d ed. (1976)

Viessmann, Warren, Introduction to Hydrology, 2d ed. (1977)

Vohora, S. B. (1981): *Is the Human Body a Microcosm? - A Critical study.* Studies Hist. Med.5 (1), 61

Wagner, A. F., and Folkers, Karl, *Vitamins and Coenzymes* (1964)

Wainwright, S. D., *Control Mechanism and Protein Synthesis* (1972)

Watson, James D., Molecular Biology of the Gene, 3d ed. (1976)

Weinstein, Boris, ed., Chemistry and Biochemistry of Amino Acids, Peptides, and Proteins, 7 vols. (1974-83)

Weissbach, Herbert, and Pestka, Sidney, eds., Molecular Mechanism of Protein Biosynthesis (1977)

White, Benjamin, Silver: Its History and Romance (1920

Wilbur, Charles C., Selenium (1983)

William Morrow & Co.; *Silver our Mightiest Germ Fighter,* Scientist Digest, March 1978

Winter, Ruth, A Consumer's Dictionary of Food Additives, rev. ed. (1984)

Wynn, Colin H., *The Structure and Function of Enzymes* (1974)

Young, A. S., *Sulfur Dioxide, Chlorine, Fluorine and Chlorine Oxides* (1983)

Zeffren, Eugene, and Hall, P. L., *The Study of Enzyme Mechanisms* (1973)

Zingaro, R. A., and Cooper, W. C., Selenium (1974)